Atlas of Electromyography

ATLAS OF
ELECTROMYOGRAPHY

A. ARTURO LEIS, M.D.

Professor of Neurology
University of Mississippi Medical Center
Mississippi Methodist Rehabilitation Center
Jackson, Mississippi

VICENTE C. TRAPANI, M.D.

Neurology Resident
University of Mississippi Medical Center
Jackson, Mississippi

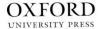

OXFORD
UNIVERSITY PRESS

2000

OXFORD
UNIVERSITY PRESS

Oxford   New York
Athens   Auckland   Bangkok   Bogotá   Buenos Aires   Calcutta
Cape Town   Chennai   Dar es Salaam   Delhi   Florence   Hong Kong   Istanbul
Karachi   Kuala Lumpur   Madrid   Melbourne   Mexico City   Mumbai
Nairobi   Paris   São Paulo   Singapore   Taipei   Tokyo   Toronto   Warsaw

and associated companies in
Berlin   Ibadan

Published by Oxford University Press, Inc.,
198 Madison Avenue, New York, New York 10016

Oxford is a registered trademark of Oxford University Press

Library of Congress Cataloging-in-Publication Data
Leis, A. Arturo.
Atlas of electromyography / A. Arturo Leis, Vicente C. Trapani.
p.   cm.
ISBN 0–19–511250–4
1. Electromyography Atlases.
I. Trapani, Vicente C.   II. Title.
[DNLM: 1. Electromyography Atlases.   2. Anatomy, Regional Atlases.
3. Muscles—innervation Atlases.
WE 17 L532a 2000]   RC77.5.L45   2000   616.7'407547—dc21
DNLM/DLC   for Library of Congress   99–15580

9 8 7 6 5 4 3

Printed in the United States of America
on acid-free paper

To my wife Donna,
for her love and support,
and to my parents,
Drs. José and Bertha Leis,
who taught me the value of an education.
A.A.L.

To my beautiful daughter Gabrielle,
to Clare McCarthy with
deep appreciation and love,
and to my parents
Corrado and Irma Trapani,
who encouraged and guided me
in my studies.
V.C.T.

Foreword

It is with pleasure that I prepare this foreword to a work from a colleague whose professional accomplishments I have followed closely for the past ten years. Indeed, as one of his mentors during his fellowship years at the University of Iowa, I have witnessed firsthand Dr. Leis' proficiency in clinical neurophysiology and his insatiable desire to learn and to teach. Early on, that desire culminated in the American Association of Electrodiagnostic Medicine's (AAEM) Golseth Award.

Dr. Leis' scientific accomplishments in the areas of motor control and clinical neurophysiology have subsequently propelled him to the rank of professor of neurology at the University of Mississippi Medical Center. His scientific accomplishments have not overshadowed his desire to educate a new generation of clinical neurophysiologists. He has received numerous Teacher of the Year Awards, which no doubt reflect his priority of educating residents and fellows, and his ability to simplify even complex problems. I believe Dr. Leis' passion for teaching is reflected in this atlas of electromyography.

The beginner will enjoy the visually alluring anatomical illustrations and the corresponding human photographs that serve as a simple guide to muscle localization. Clinical comments pertinent to the muscle of interest will help to ease the beginner's anxiety about the needle examination. The more experienced electromyographer will appreciate the well-organized, practical outlines of clinical conditions and entrapment syndromes that include lists of the etiologies, clinical features, and electrodiagnostic strategies. Both novice and expert will benefit from the numerous aids to the examination of the peripheral nervous system.

I take great pride in knowing that this atlas is the product of one of our former students. This book meets the practical needs of physicians who perform the art of electromyography and provides a commonsense approach to problem solving for frequently encountered neuromuscular lesions. I have no doubt that the atlas will be widely used by residents, fellows, and practitioners, and that it will become a standard guide in electromyography. I hope that its use will not only enhance the electromyographic evaluation, but also encourage research in the field of electrodiagnostic medicine.

Jun Kimura, M.D.
Professor Emeritus
Kyoto University, Kyoto
Professor
Department of Neurology
University of Iowa Hospitals and Clinics
Iowa City, Iowa

Preface

The seed for this book was planted by a second-year resident in Neurology, Vicente ("Enzo") Trapani, who desired a handbook in electromyography (EMG) that emphasized both muscle localization and clinical pearls. A gifted artist, Trapani envisioned a text that would provide high-quality illustrations of skeletal muscles that included nerve, plexus, and root supply; photographs of each muscle in a healthy subject to identify optimum site of EMG needle insertion; clinical features of the major conditions affecting peripheral nerves; and electrodiagnostic strategies for confirming suspected lesions of the peripheral nervous system.

The book was also nurtured by my personal experience as a program director in Clinical Neurophysiology. Many residents and fellows offered encouragement and constructive criticism. This added further incentive to improve the content and style and to make it more useful for trainees in neurology and physical medicine and rehabilitation programs. This book should be of value to these trainees and to practicing electromyographers regardless of their clinical disciplines. The book also provides numerous aids to the examination of the peripheral nervous system, which should prove useful to members of other specialties, including critical care medicine, neurological surgery, and family practice. The general practitioner may also choose to use this book as an anatomical guide.

Many of the anatomical and clinical descriptions contained in this book are derived from reviews of several editions of Gray's Anatomy as well as Sunderland's writings on peripheral nerves and nerve injuries. Additionally, publications by the American Association of Electrodiagnostic Medicine proved invaluable. Therefore, this book should ideally be used in conjunction with these other sources.

The book is divided into sections based on the major peripheral nerves. Each nerve is illustrated, and its anatomy is reviewed in the text. This is followed by a detailed outline of the clinical conditions and entrapment syndromes that affect the nerve, including a list of the etiologies, clinical features, and electrodiagnostic strategies used for each syndrome. General comments about the syndrome are also provided. Finally, each muscle supplied by the peripheral nerve is shown in an anatomical illustration and in a corresponding human photograph. The illustration shows the root, plexus, and peripheral nerve supply to the muscle. Written text provides information about the muscle origin, tendon insertion, voluntary activation maneuver, and site of optimum needle insertion. The latter is identified by a black dot (or sometimes a needle electrode) in both the anatomical illustration and the corresponding human photograph. This ensures that pertinent bony, muscular, and soft tissue landmarks can be used to guide the electromyographer to a specific point on the skin for needle insertion. Potential pitfalls associated with the needle insertion are pointed out—usually adjacent muscles or structures that may be entered by mistake. Clinical correlates pertinent to the muscle being examined are also added.

I hope that use of this book will promote interest and research in peripheral neuroanatomy and electrodiagnostic medicine.

University of Mississippi Medical Center
Jackson, Miss.   A.A.L.

Acknowledgments

We are grateful to Michael P. Schenk, CMI (Director), Richard J. Manning and Diane F. Johnson (staff), Medical Illustration Department, University of Mississippi Medical Center; and Robert Waldo Gray and Charles P. Runyan, Medical Photography Department, University of Mississippi Medical Center. We thank Mary Mann Austin, Alfredo Gomez, and Melissa Grimes for serving as models for some of the photographs. We also owe gratitude to Melissa Grimes, Chief Electromyography Technologist, for her technical and administrative assistance in preparing this book.

I (A. Leis) am indebted to Jun Kimura, M.D., for teaching me the principles and practice of electromyography, and to my colleagues in the Department of Neurology at the University of Mississippi Medical Center for doing the "busy" work while I devoted myself to writing. Special thanks go to Mark A. Ross, M.D., and Mark S. Talamonti, M.D. for their encouragement and friendship.

I (V. Trapani) wish to extend my thanks to Drs. M. Shamsnia, L. Weisberg, S. Palliyeth, and D. Schlossberg for helping and supporting me prior to my neurology training.

Contents

Atlas of Electromyography

chapter

1

Brachial

Plexus

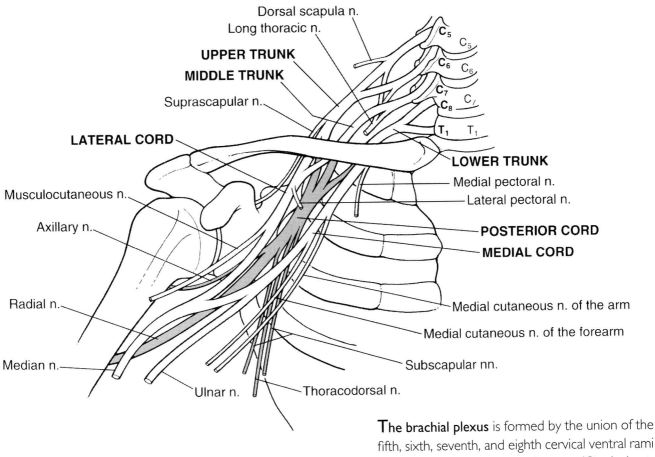

Diagram of the brachial plexus (anterior view)
and its branches.

The brachial plexus is formed by the union of the
fifth, sixth, seventh, and eighth cervical ventral rami
and the first thoracic ventral ramus (Gray's Anatomy, 1995). Contributions to the plexus from C_4
and T_2 vary. In a *prefixed* plexus, the contribution
from C_4 is large and the branch from T_1 is reduced.
In a *postfixed* plexus, the contribution from T_2 is
large and the branch from C_5 is reduced. In the
most common arrangement, the C_5 and C_6 rami

unite at the lateral border of the scalenus medius to form the *upper trunk*, C_7 gives rise to the *middle trunk*, and C_8 and T_1 join behind the scalenus anterior as the *lower trunk*. The three trunks descend laterally; at the level of the clavicle each trunk bifurcates into anterior and posterior divisions. The anterior divisions of the upper and middle trunks form the *lateral cord*, lateral to the axillary artery. The anterior division of the lower trunk emerges medial to the axillary artery to form the *medial cord*, which may also receive a branch from the C_7 ramus. Posterior divisions of all three trunks form the *posterior cord*, posterior to the axillary artery.

Brachial plexus lesions may involve the entire plexus or be confined to a particular part of it; the degree of nerve injury is seldom uniform. Acute lesions of the brachial plexus may be due to open or closed injury. In open injuries, wounding is commonly due to gun shot or sharp penetrating objects and involves the more superficial part of the plexus. Wounding involving the lower plexus is more likely to be fatal because of simultaneous damage to the lung and great vessels at the root of the neck (Sunderland, 1968). In closed injuries the causative agent is commonly traction or compression of the plexus. Neuralgic amyotrophy, also known as idiopathic brachial plexopathy, Parsonage-Turner syndrome, shoulder girdle neuritis, or acute brachial neuropathy, ranks first in incidence among nontraumatic conditions (Beghi et al., 1985), and most commonly affects the upper plexus and shoulder girdle muscles (Subramony, 1988).

UPPER TRUNK LESION

Etiology
Neuralgic amyotrophy is the most common nontraumatic condition and usually affects the upper plexus and shoulder girdle muscles.

Trauma, including stab or gunshot wounds.

Stretch injuries occur when the neck and shoulder are violently forced apart, when a blow or heavy weight depresses the shoulder, or when an adducted limb is forced violently downward (Sunderland, 1968). Stretch injuries include traction injury during difficult delivery (birth palsy), "rucksack" or "pack palsy" due to lifting a heavy backpack, and the football injury known as a "stinger" (Kimura, 1989).

General Comments
Stretch injuries to the upper trunk may be combined with C_5, C_6 root avulsion (Erb's palsy).

Clinical Features
The distribution of weakness is similar to that of Erb's palsy, with involvement of the shoulder and upper arm and sparing of hand function.

There is gross wasting of shoulder girdle muscles with a complete inability to abduct or externally rotate the arm and marked weakness of elbow flexion and radial wrist extension.

Numbness occurs over the lateral aspects of the arm, forearm, and hand.

The biceps stretch reflex is absent or reduced.

Electrodiagnostic Strategy

Use nerve conduction studies to confirm a lesion of the upper trunk (low amplitude or unelicitable sensory responses from superficial radial, lateral cutaneous nerve of forearm and median nerve recording from thumb or index finger; low amplitude or unelicitable motor responses from biceps and deltoid). In a predominantly demyelinating lesion, routine nerve conduction studies may be normal; search for local demyelinating block or slowing of conduction across the site of injury. Note: Sensory responses are normal in radiculopathies because the lesion is proximal to the dorsal root ganglion (preganglionic lesion) and the cell bodies in the ganglion maintain viability of the peripheral sensory fiber.

Demonstrate neurogenic electromyography (EMG) needle examination (i.e., spontaneous activity, abnormal motor unit potentials, abnormal recruitment) in muscles supplied by the upper trunk.

Use needle EMG to exclude C_5, C_6 radiculopathies. Radiculopathies may produce neurogenic findings in paraspinal muscles as well as limb muscles; plexopathies never do so because the plexus is formed by *ventral rami*, whereas paraspinal muscles are innervated by *posterior rami* (Wilbourn, 1985).

MIDDLE TRUNK LESION

Etiology

Neuralgic amyotrophy is a nontraumatic cause.

Isolated injury to the middle trunk is rare.

With lateral traction on the arm, the middle trunk may be the first to be injured (Sunderland, 1968).

General Comments

The middle trunk occupies a position between upper and lower trunks, being at times damaged with either the upper plexus or the lower plexus.

Clinical Features

Weakness occurs in the general territory of the radial nerve, with partial involvement of the triceps and other C_7-innervated muscles and sparing of brachioradialis.

Numbness or loss of sensation occurs in the middle finger and sometimes the index finger.

The triceps stretch reflex may be reduced.

Electrodiagnostic Strategy

Nerve conduction studies may suggest a lesion of the middle trunk (low amplitude or unelicitable sensory responses from median nerve–innervated middle finger and possibly index finger; the remaining studies are normal). In a demyelinating lesion, routine nerve conduction studies may be normal; search for local demyelinating block or slowing of conduction across the site of injury. Note: Sensory responses are normal in a C_7 radiculopathy because the lesion is proximal to the dorsal root ganglion (preganglionic lesion) and the cell bodies in the ganglion maintain viability of the peripheral sensory fibers.

Demonstrate neurogenic EMG needle examination (i.e., spontaneous activity, abnormal motor unit potentials, abnormal recruitment) in muscles supplied by the middle trunk.

Use needle EMG to exclude C_7 radiculopathy. Radiculopathies may produce neurogenic EMG in paraspinal muscles as well as limb muscles; plexopathies never do so because the plexus is formed by *ventral rami*, whereas paraspinal muscles are innervated by *posterior rami* (Wilbourn, 1985).

LOWER TRUNK LESION

Etiology

Metastasis (lymph node infiltration in axilla) or direct invasion (Pancoast's tumor in apex of lung) can cause a lower trunk lesion.

Neuralgic amyotrophy is a nontraumatic cause.

Neurogenic thoracic outlet syndrome (TOS) is a rare cause.

Traumatic causes include stab wounds and bullet wounds.

Traction applied to the fully abducted arm (i.e., subject jerked upward by the outstretched arm) can cause a lower trunk lesion.

General Comments

True neurogenic TOS is rare (1 per 1,000,000) and results from lower trunk fibers being stretched over a fibrous band extending from the first rib to the C_7 transverse process or a rudimentary cervical rib (Wilbourn, 1988).

When traction is applied to the fully abducted arm, it is the lower roots and trunk of the plexus that suffer most (Sunderland, 1968).

Stretch injuries to the lower trunk may be combined with C_8, T_1 root avulsion (Klumpke's palsy).

Clinical Features

The distribution of weakness is similar to that of Klumpke's palsy, with involvement of all intrinsic hand muscles and sparing of shoulder and upper arm muscles.

In addition to intrinsic hand muscles, finger flexors and extensors in the forearm are weak.

Numbness or loss of sensation occurs in the medial aspect of the arm, medial forearm, and medial hand, including fourth and fifth digits.

Electrodiagnostic Strategy

Use nerve conduction studies to localize a lesion to the lower trunk or medial cord (low amplitude or unelicitable sensory responses from little finger and medial cutaneous nerve of forearm; low amplitude or unelicitable motor responses from median and ulnar hand muscles). In a demyelinating lesion, special nerve conduction studies may be needed to demonstrate demyelinating block or slowing of conduction across the site of injury. Note: Sensory responses are normal in radiculopathies because the lesion is proximal to the dorsal root ganglion.

Demonstrate neurogenic EMG needle examination (i.e., spontaneous activity, abnormal motor unit potentials, abnormal recruitment) in muscles supplied by the lower trunk.

Exclude C_8, T_1 radiculopathies by needle EMG. Radiculopathies may produce neurogenic EMG in paraspinal muscles as well as limb muscles; plexopathies never do so because the plexus is formed by *ventral rami*, whereas paraspinal muscles are innervated by *posterior rami* (Wilbourn, 1985).

CORD LESIONS

General Comments

The consequences of lesions affecting the lateral, medial, or posterior cords of the brachial plexus may be determined by combining the effects following injury to the individual nerves that originate from the respective cords (Sunderland, 1968).

REFERENCES

Beghi E, Kurland L T, Mulder D W, Nicolosi A. Brachial plexus neuropathy in the population of Rochester, Minnesota, 1970–1981. Ann Neurol 1985; 18:320–323.

Gray's Anatomy. 38th Edition. Churchill Livingstone, New York, 1995, pp 1266–1274.

Kimura J. Electrodiagnosis in Diseases of Nerve And Muscle. 2nd Edition. F A Davis, Philadelphia, 1989, pp 447–461.

Subramony S H. AAEE case report #14: Neuralgic amyotrophy (acute brachial neuropathy). Muscle Nerve 1988; 11:39–44.

Sunderland S. Nerves and Nerve Injuries. Williams & Wilkins, Baltimore, 1968, pp 953–1011.

Wilbourn A J. Electrodiagnosis of plexopathies. Neurol Clin 1985; 3:511–529.

Wilbourn A J. Thoracic outlet syndrome surgery causing severe brachial plexopathy. Muscle Nerve 1988; 11:66–74.

chapter
2

Median

Nerve

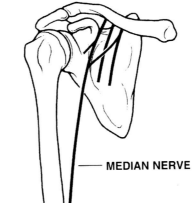

— **MEDIAN NERVE**

Pronator teres
Flexor carpi radialis
Palmaris longus
Flexor digitorum superficialis

**ANTERIOR
INTEROSSEOUS
NERVE**

Flexor digitorum profundus

Flexor pollicis longus

Pronator quadratus

Abductor pollicis brevis
Flexor pollicis brevis
Opponens pollicis

First lumbrical
Second lumbrical

Diagram of the median nerve and the muscles that it supplies. Note: The white oval signifies that a muscle receives a part of its innervation from another peripheral nerve.

The median nerve is formed in the axilla from the medial and lateral cords of the brachial plexus. The lateral cord conveys fibers from the fifth, sixth, and seventh cervical spinal nerves, while the medial cord supplies fibers from the eighth cervical and first thoracic spinal nerves (Gray's Anatomy, 1995). The median nerve innervates no muscles in the upper arm. In the cubital fossa, the nerve is accompanied by the brachial artery, which divides into radial and ulnar arteries at the neck of the radius. From this position, the nerve continues distally between the two heads of the pronator teres to reach the forearm proper. It supplies the pronator teres, flexor carpi radialis, palmaris longus, and flexor digitorum superficialis. It then gives rise to a pure motor branch, the *anterior interosseous nerve,* which innervates the flexor digitorum profundus to digits 2 and 3, flexor pollicis longus, and pronator quadratus. The nerve then descends the forearm and passes through the carpal tunnel as it enters the palm. It supplies the first and second lumbricals and gives off the recurrent thenar branch to the abductor pollicis brevis, flexor pollicis brevis (superficial head), and opponens pollicis. The median nerve also subserves sensation to the skin overlying the lateral aspect of the palm, dorsal surface of the distal phalanges, volar surface of the thumb, index and middle fingers, and half of the ring finger.

Although the median nerve, or its branches, may be affected by penetrating injuries at any level, there are certain sites where the nerve is prone to injury (Sunderland, 1968). In the upper arm, the nerve is closely bound to the axillary artery and then to the brachial artery as far as the cubital fossa. This close relationship explains why combined nerve–arterial injury is common in this region and why the nerve is subject to compression from aneurysms. In the lower arm, a spur of bone may rarely project from the anteromedial aspect of the supracondylar surface of the humerus and be joined to the medial epicondyle by a strong ligament (Struther's ligament). This ligament may compress the median nerve proximal to the innervation to the pronator teres. In the pronator teres syndrome, the median nerve is injured in the upper forearm due to trauma, fracture, or, under exceptional circumstances, compression between the two heads of the pronator teres or a fibrous band as it emerges from this muscle. More distally in the forearm, the anterior interosseous branch may be injured by trauma or as a consequence of neuralgic amyotrophy. Entrapment of the anterior interosseous nerve may also result from fibrous bands or anomalous muscles (Wertsch, 1992). At the wrist, damage to the median nerve is commonly due to compression of the nerve in the carpal tunnel. This results in *carpal tunnel syndrome,* the most common entrapment neuropathy in humans.

CARPAL TUNNEL SYNDROME

Etiology
Carpal tunnel syndrome is caused by compression of the nerve in the carpal tunnel.

General Comments
Carpal tunnel syndrome is the most common entrapment neuropathy.
Women are affected more often than men.
Symptoms usually involve the dominant hand, with a higher incidence in persons who use their hands occupationally.
Predisposing conditions include obesity, pregnancy, polyneuropathy, diabetes, amyloidosis, acromegaly, rheumatoid arthritis, myxedema, and lupus erythematosus.

Clinical Features
Hand pain may be perceived more proximally in the forearm, arm, or shoulder, mimicking cervical radiculopathy.

Numbness usually involves the lateral four digits, but all digits may be affected or sensory loss may be confined to one digit.

Pain and paresthesia are aggravated by repetitive use of the hand.

Patients characteristically awaken at night with symptoms (nocturnal paresthesia).

In severe cases, there is weakness and atrophy of thenar muscles.

Onset is insidious in most cases.

Electrodiagnostic Strategy

Use nerve conduction studies to confirm a focal lesion of median sensory and motor fibers in the carpal tunnel. Many techniques have been developed for identifying conduction abnormalities within the carpal tunnel (Ross and Kimura, 1995).

Perform EMG needle examination in thenar muscles. In carpal tunnel syndrome associated with loss of motor fibers, EMG will show neurogenic changes (i.e., spontaneous activity, abnormal motor unit potentials, abnormal recruitment).

If EMG of thenar muscles is abnormal, study proximal median-innervated muscles to exclude median nerve lesion above the wrist. Also, study C_8, T_1 muscles innervated by ulnar or radial nerves to exclude C_8, T_1 radiculopathy.

If clinical symptoms or signs suggest cervical radiculopathy, study muscles supplied by C_6 and C_7 roots to exclude C_6 or C_7 radiculopathy. The differential diagnosis for carpal tunnel syndrome includes C_6 and C_7 radiculopathies due to overlap of dermatomes with median sensory distribution.

ANTERIOR INTEROSSEOUS NERVE SYNDROME

Etiology

Neuralgic amyotrophy (idiopathic brachial plexopathy) may exclusively affect the anterior interosseous nerve (AIN).

Trauma, including stab wounds and gunshot wounds, can cause AIN syndrome.

Entrapment may rarely result from fibrous bands or anomalous muscles (Wertsch, 1992).

General Comments

The AIN is the largest branch of the median nerve.

It is a "pure" motor nerve because it lacks a cutaneous representation. However, sensory fibers from wrist and hand joints travel in the AIN.

The AIN innervates three muscles: flexor digitorum profundus (digits 2 and 3), flexor pollicis longus, and pronator quadratus.

Fifty percent of Martin-Gruber anastomoses arise from the AIN.

Clinical Features

A typical symptom is acute onset of thumb and index finger weakness.

Numbness and tingling do not occur.

A dull, aching pain may be present in the volar wrist or forearm.

The patient is unable to form an "O" with the thumb and index finger (due to weak flexion of terminal phalanges of the thumb and index finger).

Weakness in the pronator quadratus may be difficult to detect.

In a person with Martin-Gruber anastomosis and AIN syndrome, there may be additional weakness or atrophy of intrinsic hand muscles supplied by the crossing fibers (Wertsch, 1992).

The cutaneous sensory examination is normal.

Electrodiagnostic Strategy

Routine nerve conduction studies are normal.

Perform EMG needle examination in multiple muscles, including proximal and scapular muscles. EMG is crucial for identifying the possibility that AIN syndrome is a manifestation of neuralgic amyotrophy.

In AIN syndrome, EMG will show neurogenic changes (spontaneous activity, abnormal motor unit potentials, abnormal recruitment) in the flexor digitorum profundus to digits 2 and 3, flexor pollicis longus, and pronator quadratus.

In a person with Martin-Gruber anastomosis and AIN syndrome, EMG may show neurogenic changes in muscles supplied by the crossing fibers (usually dorsal interossei, adductor pollicis, or abductor digiti minimi).

PRONATOR TERES SYNDROME

Etiology

Trauma, usually deep penetrating wounds, is causative.

Entrapment occurs between the two heads of the pronator teres or by a fibrous band connecting the pronator teres with the tendinous arch of the flexor digitorum superficialis.

General Comments

Some investigators have never encountered a true entrapment of the median nerve as it passes through the pronator teres; there is some doubt as to whether such an entrapment exists.

Clinical Features

Pain and tenderness occur over the pronator teres.

Numbness or tingling can occur in the median sensory distribution of the hand, including over the proximal palm and thenar eminence. (Note: The palmar cutaneous branch is spared in carpal tunnel syndrome because it passes superficial to the carpal tunnel. Sensory deficits in the palm and thenar eminence can help to differentiate pronator teres syndrome from carpal tunnel syndrome.)

In severe cases, there is weakness and atrophy of the median innervated muscles distal to the pronator teres.

Electrodiagnostic Strategy

Nerve conduction studies may show reduced conduction velocity or conduction block in the median nerve in the elbow to wrist segment.

EMG may show a neurogenic pattern in median-innervated muscles distal to the pronator teres.

LIGAMENT OF STRUTHER'S SYNDROME

Etiology

Entrapment is caused by Struther's ligament, which is a fibrous band joining the supracondylar process (bony spur) on the anteromedial aspect of the lower humerus with the medial epicondyle of the humerus.

General Comments

A supracondylar process is present in only 0.3%–2.7% of humans (Pecina et al., 1997). When the supracondylar process is present, the median nerve and sometimes the brachial artery deviates medially to pass under Struther's ligament.

Clinical Features

Pain and paresthesia occur in the median sensory distribution of the hand, including the palm and thenar eminence (Note: The palmar cutaneous branch is spared in the carpal tunnel syndrome because it passes superficial to the carpal tunnel.)

In severe cases, there is weakness and atrophy of all median-innervated muscles, including the pronator teres. Weakness of pronation differentiates this condition from pronator teres syndrome.

Radiographic studies (plain films) show the supracondylar bony spur.

Electrodiagnostic Strategy

Nerve conduction studies may show reduced conduction velocity or conduction block in the median nerve in the upper arm to elbow segment.

Demonstrate neurogenic EMG in the median-innervated muscles, including the pronator teres.

REFERENCES

Bergman R A, Thompson S A, Afifi A K. Catalog of Human Variation. Urban & Schwarzenberg, Baltimore, 1984, pp 31–32.

Gray's Anatomy. 38th Edition, Churchill Livingstone, New York, 1995, pp 1266–1274.

Pecina M M, Krmpotic-Nemanic J, Markiewitz, A D. Tunnel Syndromes: Peripheral Nerve Compression Syndromes. 2nd Edition. CRC Press, New York, 1997, pp 73–76.

Ross M A, Kimura J. AAEM case report #2: The carpal tunnel syndrome. Muscle Nerve 1995; 18: 567–573.

Sunderland S. Nerves and Nerve Injuries. Williams & Wilkins, Baltimore, 1968, pp 781–807.

Wertsch J J. AAEM case report #25: Anterior interosseous nerve syndrome. Muscle Nerve 1992; 15: 977–983.

Abductor Pollicis Brevis

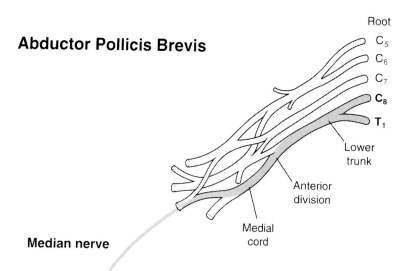

Median nerve

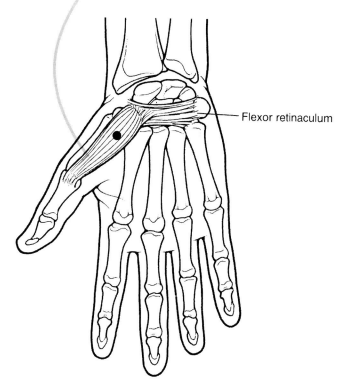

Flexor retinaculum

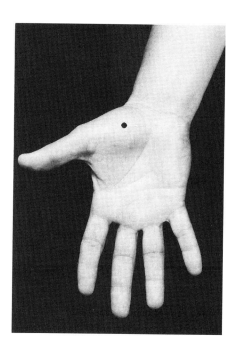

Innervation
Innervation is via the median nerve, medial cord, lower trunk, and roots C_8, T_1.

Origin
The muscle originates in the palmar retinaculum and the tubercle of the scaphoid and trapezium.

Insertion
The muscle is inserted at the base of the proximal phalanx of the thumb.

Activation Maneuver
Abduction of the thumb (movement of the thumb out of the plane of the palm) activates the muscle.

EMG Needle Insertion
Insert the needle obliquely near the muscle origin. Assess abnormal EMG activity by directing the needle distally along the muscle.

Pitfalls
If the needle is inserted too medially, it may penetrate the flexor pollicis brevis, which receives dual innervation from the median and ulnar nerves.

If the needle is inserted too deeply, it may penetrate the adductor pollicis, which receives innervation from the ulnar nerve.

Clinical Comments
Needle examination may show neurogenic changes with axonal loss lesions of the median nerve due to carpal tunnel syndrome, pronator teres syndrome, ligament of Struther's syndrome, medial cord lesions, C_8, T_1 radiculopathy, Klumpke's palsy (C_8, T_1 root avulsion), and anterior horn cell disease.

EMG will be normal in the anterior interosseous nerve syndrome.

Opponens Pollicis

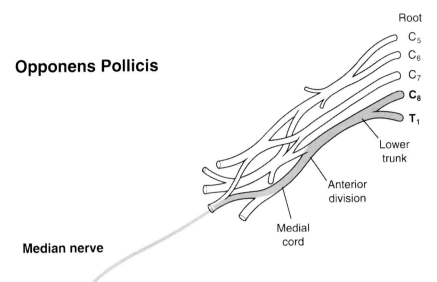

Root
C₅
C₆
C₇
C₈
T₁

Lower trunk

Anterior division

Medial cord

Median nerve

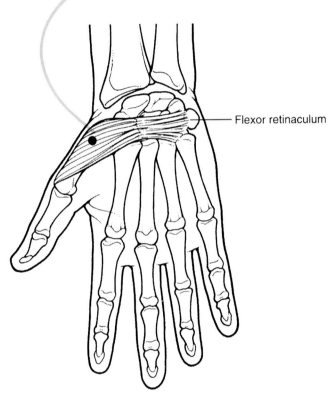

Flexor retinaculum

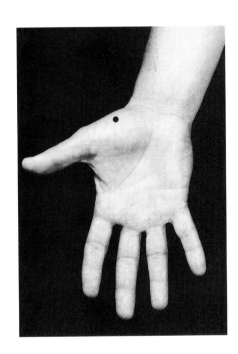

Innervation
Innervation is via the median nerve, medial cord, lower trunk, and roots C_8, T_1.

Origin
The muscle originates in the palmar retinaculum, and the tubercle of the trapezium.

Insertion
The muscle is inserted at the palmar surface of the first metacarpal bone.

Activation Maneuver
Opposition of the thumb to the little finger activates the muscle.

EMG Needle Insertion
Insert the needle obliquely at the midpoint of the first metacarpal shaft just lateral to the abductor pollicis brevis muscle.

Pitfalls
If the needle is inserted too medially, it will be in the abductor pollicis brevis, which still receives innervation from the median nerve. If inserted even more medially, it may be in the flexor pollicis brevis, which receives dual innervation from the median and ulnar nerves. If the needle is inserted too deeply, it may penetrate the adductor pollicis, which receives innervation from the ulnar nerve.

Clinical Comments
EMG may show neurogenic changes in the carpal tunnel syndrome, pronator teres syndrome, ligament of Struther's syndrome, medial cord lesions, C_8, T_1 radiculopathy, Klumpke's palsy (C_8, T_1 root avulsion), and anterior horn cell disease.
EMG will be normal in the anterior interosseous nerve syndrome.

Flexor Pollicis Brevis

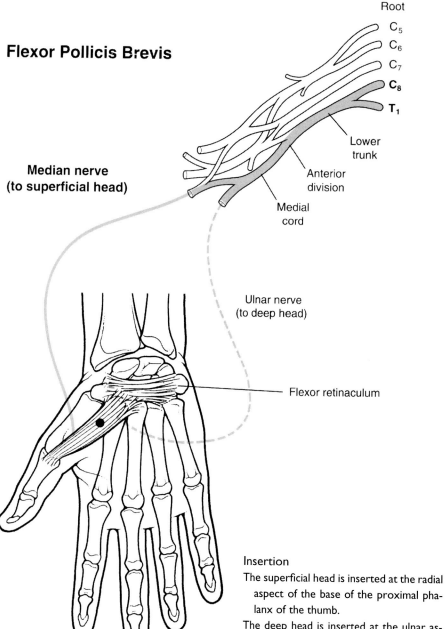

Root
C₅
C₆
C₇
C₈
T₁

Lower trunk

Median nerve (to superficial head)

Anterior division

Medial cord

Ulnar nerve (to deep head)

Flexor retinaculum

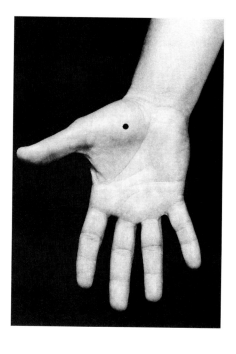

Innervation
Superficial head: Innervation is via the median nerve, medial cord, lower trunk, and roots C_8, T_1.
Deep head: Innervation is via the ulnar nerve, medial cord, lower trunk, and roots C_8, T_1.

Origin
The superficial head originates in the flexor retinaculum and trapezium.
The deep head originates in the ulnar aspect of the first metacarpal.

Insertion
The superficial head is inserted at the radial aspect of the base of the proximal phalanx of the thumb.
The deep head is inserted at the ulnar aspect of the base of the proximal phalanx of the thumb.

Activation Maneuver
Flexing of the metacarpophalangeal joint of the thumb activates the muscle.

EMG Needle Insertion
Superficial head: Insert the needle obliquely at a depth of 0.5–1 cm at the midpoint of a line drawn between the metacarpophalangeal joint and the pisiform. Assess abnormal EMG activity by directing the needle distally along the muscle.
Deep head: The procedure is the same as that for the superficial head, but insert the needle to a depth of 1–2 cm.

Pitfalls
If the needle is inserted too deeply, it may penetrate the opponens pollicis, which is innervated by the median nerve; if inserted still deeper, it may be in the adductor pollicis, which receives innervation from the ulnar nerve.
If the needle is inserted too laterally, it will be in the abductor pollicis brevis, which receives innervation from the median nerve.

Clinical Comments
Testing of the flexor pollicis brevis is rarely of benefit in a routine EMG needle evaluation (in general, muscles that receive dual innervation should be avoided).
The superficial head will show neurogenic changes in lesions of the median nerve.
The deep head will show neurogenic changes in lesions of the ulnar nerve.
Both heads may show neurogenic changes in C_8, T_1 radiculopathy, Klumpke's palsy (C_8, T_1 root avulsion), and anterior horn cell disease.

1st, 2nd Lumbricals

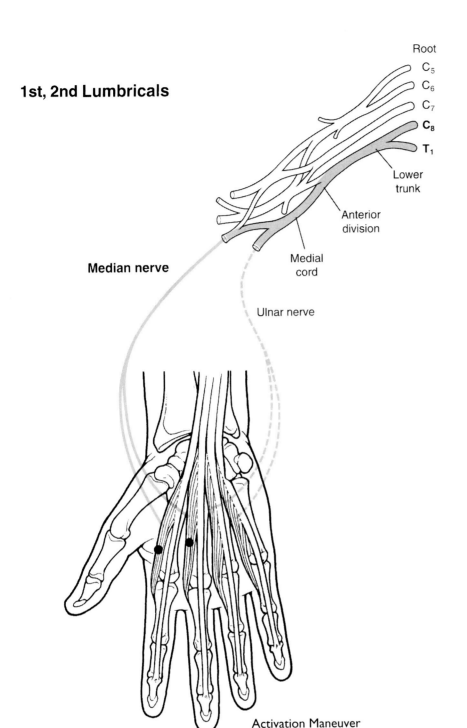

Root
C₅
C₆
C₇
C₈
T₁
Lower trunk
Anterior division
Medial cord

Median nerve

Ulnar nerve

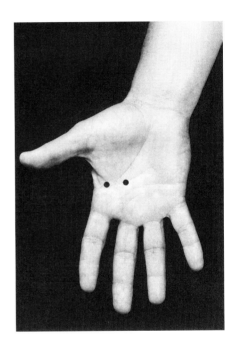

Innervation
Innervation is via the median nerve, medial cord, lower trunk, and roots C_8, T_1.

Origin
The first and second lumbricals originate in the radial aspect of the tendon sheath of the flexor digitorum profundus.

Insertion
The muscles are inserted at the radial lateral band of the dorsal digital expansion.

Activation Maneuver
Extention of the finger at the proximal interphalangeal joint with the metacarpophalangeal joint extended and fixed activates the first and second lumbricals.

EMG Needle Insertion
Insert the needle just proximal to the metacarpophalangeal joint and radial to the flexor tendon.

Pitfalls
All muscles surrounding the first and second lumbricals receive innervation from the ulnar nerve. It is therefore easy to erroneously access ulnar intrinsic hand muscles.

Clinical Comments
Lumbrical examination causes pain. It is rarely of benefit in a routine EMG needle evaluation.

Needle examination will show neurogenic changes with axonal loss lesions of median nerve due to carpal tunnel syndrome, pronator teres syndrome, ligament of Struther's syndrome, C_8, T_1 radiculopathy, Klumpke's palsy (C_8, T_1 root avulsion), and anterior horn cell disease.

Pronator Quadratus

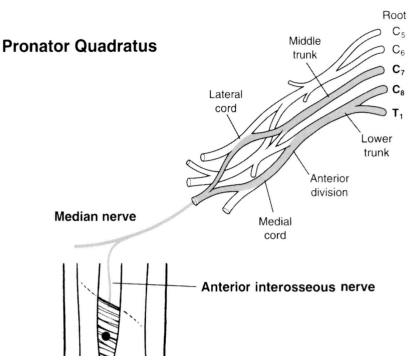

Median nerve

Anterior interosseous nerve

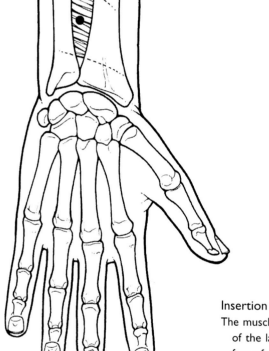

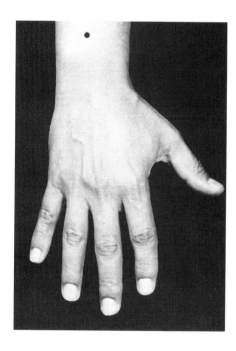

Innervation
Innervation is via the anterior interosseous branch, median nerve, lateral and medial cords, middle and lower trunks, and roots C_7, C_8, T_1.

Origin
The pronator quadratus originates in the distal fourth of the volar surface of the ulna.

Insertion
The muscle is inserted at the distal fourth of the lateral border and the volar surface of the radius.

Activation Maneuver
Pronation of the forearm activates the muscle.

EMG Needle Insertion
Place the forearm in a neutral position to full supination (this opens up the area between the ulna and the radius). Insert the needle dorsally 2–3 cm proximal to the ulnar styloid just lateral (in the radial direction) to the ulna to a depth of 2–2.5 cm. Slant the needle slightly toward the shaft of the radius to penetrate the interosseous membrane.

Pitfalls
If the needle is inserted too deeply, it may penetrate the flexor digitorum superficialis, which receives innervation from the median nerve.

Clinical Comments
EMG needle examination will be normal in the carpal tunnel syndrome.

EMG may show neurogenic changes in lesions of the anterior interosseous nerve, producing axonal loss.

EMG may show neurogenic changes in more proximal lesions affecting median nerve fibers (pronator teres syndrome, ligament of Struther's syndrome, C_7, C_8, T_1 radiculopathy, root avulsion, and anterior horn cell disease).

Flexor Pollicis Longus

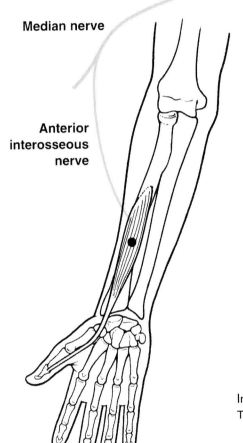

Median nerve

Anterior interosseous nerve

Root
C₅
C₆
C₇
C₈
T₁

Lateral and medial cord

Middle and lower trunk

Anterior division

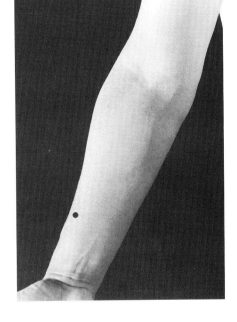

Innervation
Innervation is via the anterior interosseous branch, median nerve, lateral and medial cords, middle and lower trunks, and roots C_7, C_8, T_1.

Origin
The flexor pollicis longus originates in the volar surface of the radius.

Insertion
The muscle is inserted at the volar surface of the base of the distal phalanx of the thumb.

Activation Maneuver
Flexion of the distal phalanx of the thumb activates the flexor pollicis longus.

EMG Needle Insertion
Palpate the radial artery. Insert the needle 5–7 cm proximal and 1–1.5 cm lateral to the radial artery pulse.

Pitfalls
If the needle is inserted too superficially, it may lie in the flexor digitorum superficialis, which receives innervation from the median nerve.

If the needle is inserted too medially, the radial artery will lie in the path of the advancing needle.

Clinical Comments
EMG needle examination will be normal in the carpal tunnel syndrome.

EMG may show neurogenic changes in lesions of the anterior interosseous nerve, producing axonal loss.

EMG may show neurogenic changes in more proximal lesions affecting median nerve fibers (pronator teres syndrome, ligament of Struther's syndrome, C_7, C_8, T_1 radiculopathy, root avulsion, and anterior horn cell disease).

Flexor Digitorum Profundus
Digits 2 and 3

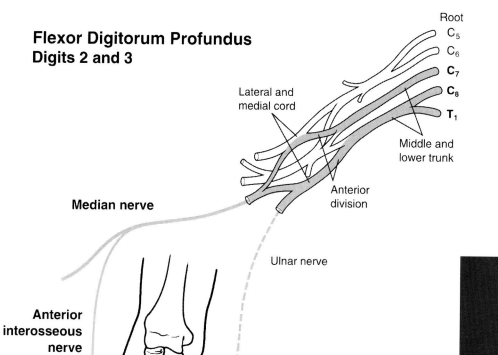

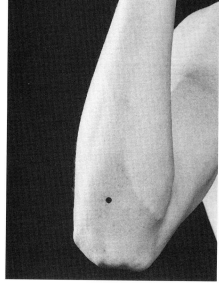

Innervation

Digits two and three: Innervation is via the anterior interosseous branch, median nerve, lateral and medial cords, middle and lower trunks, and roots C_7, C_8.

Digits four and five: Innervation is via the ulnar nerve, medial cord, lower trunk, and roots C_8, T_1.

Origin

The flexor digitorum profundus originates in the volar and medial surfaces of the ulna.

Insertion

The muscle is inserted at the volar surfaces of the bases of the distal phalanges of digits 2 through 5.

Activation Maneuver

Flexion of the distal phalanges of digits 2 through 5 activates the flexor digitorum profundus.

EMG Needle Insertion

Insert the needle 5–7 cm distal to the olecranon process and 1–1.5 cm medial to the shaft of the ulna. The ulnar innervated portion lies superficially at a depth of 1–2 cm; the median portion lies deep at a depth of 3–4 cm.

Pitfalls

If the needle is inserted too volarly (i.e., toward the palmar surface), it may lie in the flexor carpi ulnaris, which receives innervation from the ulnar nerve.

Clinical Comments

EMG of the deep portion may show neurogenic changes in the anterior interosseous nerve syndrome and in proximal lesions affecting median nerve fibers (pronator teres syndrome, ligament of Struther's syndrome, C_7, C_8 radiculopathy, avulsion, and anterior horn cell disease).

EMG of the superficial portion may show neurogenic changes in axonal loss lesions of the ulnar nerve at the elbow (cubital tunnel or retrocondylar groove).

Flexor Digitorum Superficialis (sublimis)

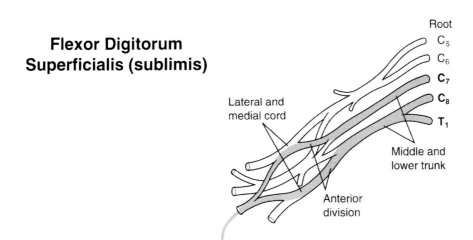

Root
C₅
C₆
C₇
C₈
T₁

Lateral and medial cord

Middle and lower trunk

Anterior division

Median nerve

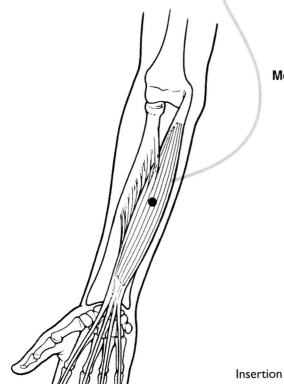

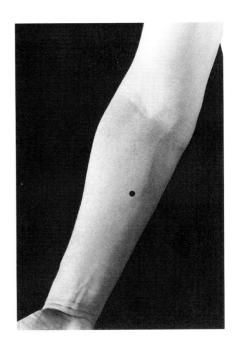

Innervation
Innervation is via the median nerve, lateral and medial cords, middle and lower trunks, and roots C_7, C_8, T_1.

Origin
The flexor digitorum superficialis (sublimis) originates in the Medial epicondyle of the humerus by the common tendon, coronoid process of ulna, and oblique line of the radius.

Insertion
Insertion is at the sides of the second phalanges of digits 2 through 5.

Activation Maneuver
Flexion of the digits at the proximal interphalangeal joint, with the proximal phalanx fixed and the distal interphalangeal joint in hyperextension, activates the muscle.

EMG Needle Insertion
Insert the needle into the volar surface of the forearm approximately 7–9 cm distal to the biceps tendon (midforearm) and 2–3 cm medial to the ventral midline.

Pitfalls
If the needle is inserted too laterally (radially), it may lie in the flexor carpi radialis, which also receives innervation from the median nerve.

If the needle is inserted too medially (ulnarly), it may be in the flexor carpi ulnaris, which receives innervation from the ulnar nerve.

If the needle is inserted too deeply, it may be in the flexor digitorum profundus (median innervated portion).

Clinical Comments
Needle examination may show neurogenic changes with axonal loss lesions of the median nerve due to pronator teres syndrome, ligament of Struther's syndrome, brachial plexopathy, C_7, C_8, or T_1 radiculopathies, and anterior horn cell disease.

Palmaris Longus

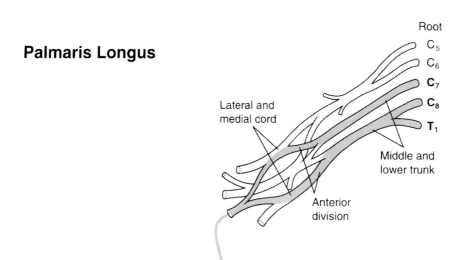

Root
C₅
C₆
C₇
C₈
T₁

Lateral and medial cord

Middle and lower trunk

Anterior division

Median nerve

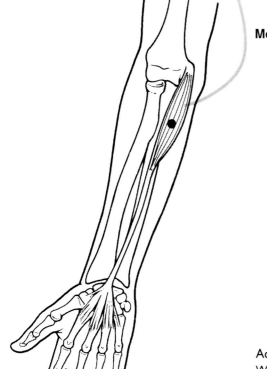

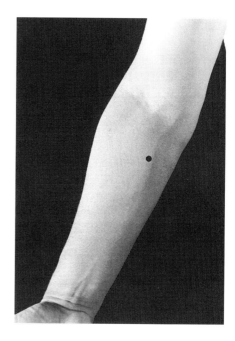

Innervation
Innervation is via the median nerve, lateral and medial cords, middle and lower trunks, and roots C_7, C_8, T_1.

Origin
The palmaris longus originates in the medial epicondyle of the humerus.

Insertion
Insertion is at the palmar aponeurosis.

Activation Maneuver
When the palm of the hand is cupped, the palmaris longus is activated.

EMG Needle Insertion
Insert the needle into the volar surface of the forearm 6–8 cm distal to the medial epicondyle along a line directed toward the muscle tendon at the wrist.

Pitfalls
If the needle is inserted too laterally (radially), it may lie in the flexor carpi radialis, which receives innervation from the median nerve.

If the needle is inserted too medially (ulnarly), it may be in the flexor carpi ulnaris, which receives innervation from the ulnar nerve.

If the needle is inserted too deeply, it may be in the flexor digitorum superficialis (median nerve innervation) or flexor digitorum profundus (median-innervated portion).

Clinical Comments
The palmaris longus is not routinely assessed. This muscle is the most variable muscle of the body (Bergman, et al., 1984). It is absent in 11% of humans (both arms in 8%; right arms, 4%; left arms, 5%).

Needle examination may show neurogenic changes with loss of axons in the median nerve due to pronator teres syndrome, ligament of Struther's syndrome, brachial plexopathy, C_7, C_8, or T_1 radiculopathies, and anterior horn cell disease.

Flexor Carpi Radialis

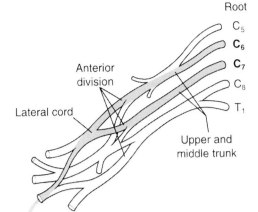

Root
C₅
C₆
C₇
C₈
T₁

Anterior division

Lateral cord

Upper and middle trunk

Median nerve

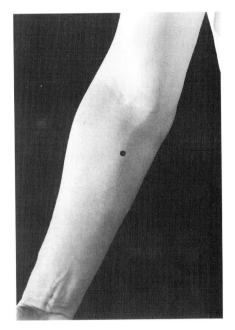

variation is partial or total attachment to the trapezium).

EMG Needle Insertion
The needle is inserted into the volar surface of the forearm 7–9 cm distal to the medial epicondyle along a line directed toward the muscle tendon at the wrist.

Activation Maneuver
Flexion of the hand at the wrist with radial deviation activates the muscle. Hint: Avoid coactivation of the flexor digitorum superficialis or the pronator teres when performing the activation maneuver.

Pitfalls
If the needle is inserted too laterally (radially), it may be in the brachioradialis (radial nerve innervation); if it is inserted too lateral and proximal, it may be in the pronator teres (median nerve innervation).

If the needle is inserted too medially (ulnarly), it may be in the flexor digitorum superficialis or palmaris longus (median nerve innervation); if inserted too deeply, it will be in the flexor digitorum superficialis (median nerve innervation).

Clinical Comments
The flexor carpi radialis is routinely examined after carpal tunnel syndrome is diagnosed to exclude coexisting proximal median nerve injury (double lesion).

Needle examination may show neurogenic changes with loss of axons in the median nerve due to pronator teres syndrome, ligament of Struther's syndrome, lateral cord lesion, C₆, C₇ radiculopathy, and anterior horn cell disease.

Innervation
Innervation is via the median nerve, lateral cord, upper and middle trunks, and roots C₆, C₇.

Origin
The flexor carpi radialis originates in the medial epicondyle of the humerus.

Insertion
Insertion is at the volar surface of the base of the second metacarpal (a common

Pronator Teres

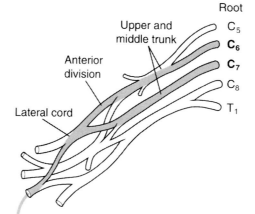

Root
C$_5$
C$_6$
C$_7$
C$_8$
T$_1$

Upper and middle trunk

Anterior division

Lateral cord

Median nerve

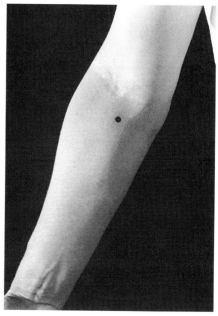

Innervation

Innervation is via the median nerve, lateral cord, upper and middle trunks, and roots C$_6$, C$_7$.

Origin

The pronator teres arises as two heads, one from the medial epicondyle of the humerus and the other from the coronoid process of the ulna.

Insertion

Insertion is at the lateral surface of the radius at the midshaft level.

EMG Needle Insertion

Insert the needle 2–3 cm distal and 1 cm medial to the biceps tendon (the edge of the muscle can be palpated in this location).

Activation Maneuver

Pronation of the forearm activates the muscle. Hint: Avoid coactivation of the flexor carpi radialis when performing the activation maneuver.

Pitfalls

If the needle is inserted too laterally (radially), it may be in the brachioradialis, which is supplied by the radial nerve.

If the needle is inserted too medially (ulnarly) or too distally, it may be in the flexor carpi radialis, which is supplied by the median nerve.

If the needle is inserted too deeply, it will be in the flexor digitorum superficialis, which is supplied by the median nerve.

Clinical Comments

The pronator teres is the most proximal muscle innervated by the median nerve.

The median nerve enters the forearm between the two heads of this muscle. Entrapment produces the pronator teres syndrome.

EMG may show neurogenic changes with loss of axons in the median nerve due to ligament of Struther's syndrome, lateral cord lesion, C$_6$, C$_7$ radiculopathy, and anterior horn cell disease.

EMG is usually normal in the pronator teres syndrome. Note: The muscle naming a syndrome is usually spared in that syndrome.

chapter
3

Ulnar

Nerve

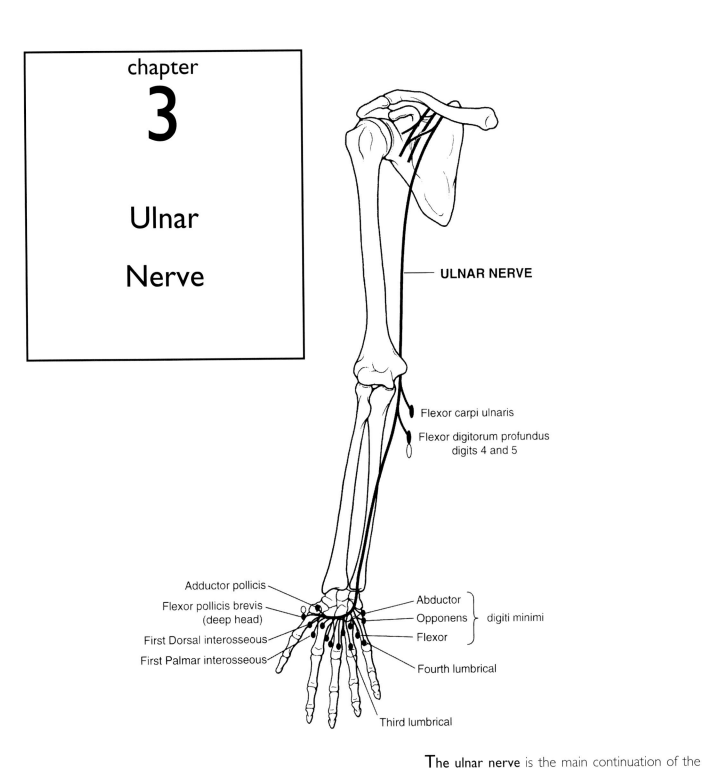

ULNAR NERVE

Flexor carpi ulnaris

Flexor digitorum profundus
digits 4 and 5

Adductor pollicis
Flexor pollicis brevis
(deep head)
First Dorsal interosseous
First Palmar interosseous

Abductor
Opponens   } digiti minimi
Flexor

Fourth lumbrical

Third lumbrical

Diagram of the ulnar nerve and the muscles that it supplies. NOTE: The white oval signifies that a muscle receives a part of its innervation from another peripheral nerve.

The ulnar nerve is the main continuation of the medial cord of the brachial plexus. Its fibers are usually derived from the eighth cervical and first thoracic roots, although occasionally the seventh cervical root makes a contribution via the lateral cord (Gray's Anatomy, 1995). In the axilla, the nerve runs between the axillary artery and vein. In the arm, it stays between the brachial artery and vein, sharing the neurovascular bundle with the median nerve. At the midarm, it leaves the neurovascular bundle and passes posteriorly through the medial intermuscular septum to descend on the medial aspect of the medial head of the triceps. The nerve is superficial throughout this course and innervates no muscles in the arm.

At the elbow, the nerve lies in a groove formed by the medial epicondyle of the humerus and the olecranon process of the ulna (the retrocondylar groove). It enters the forearm through an aponeurotic arcade (the cubital tunnel) joining the two heads of the flexor carpi ulnaris, which it innervates. The arcade typically lies about 1.5 cm distal to the medial epicondyle (Campbell, 1989). The nerve travels through the belly of the flexor carpi ulnaris and then exits by piercing the aponeurosis on the undersurface of the muscle. It then lies in the plane between the flexor carpi ulnaris and the flexor digitorum profundus (to digits 4 and 5), which it innervates.

The nerve is joined by the ulnar artery in the upper forearm to form a neurovascular bundle. About the middle of the forearm, the ulnar nerve gives rise to the palmar cutaneous branch, which descends to provide sensory innervation to the medial aspect of the proximal palm. About 7 cm proximal to the wrist it also gives off a dorsal cutaneous branch, which provides innervation to the medial aspect of the dorsum of the hand and the dorsoproximal aspect of the fifth and medial fourth digits. The ulnar nerve provides no sensory innervation above the wrist. Hence, sensory loss in the forearm or arm is not a feature of an ulnar nerve lesion.

At the wrist, the ulnar nerve and artery lie in a canal formed by the pisiform medially and the hook of the hamate laterally (Guyon's canal). In this region the nerve divides into superficial and deep branches. Although the superficial branch is generally considered a sensory branch, it supplies the palmaris brevis, a thin muscle beneath the skin of the proximal medial palm, which cannot be studied electromyographically. It then provides sensory innervation to the distal palm and terminates in two digital branches that are distributed to the ulnar side of the fifth digit and the adjoining sides of the fourth and fifth digits. The deep muscular branch gives off a hypothenar branch to innervate the abductor, opponens, and flexor digit minimi. It then follows the course of the deep palmar arch across the hand. As it crosses, it supplies dorsal and palmar interossei and the third and fourth lumbricals. At its termination between the thumb and index fingers, it supplies the flexor pollicis brevis (deep head) and adductor pollicis.

Although the ulnar nerve, or its branches, may be involved by penetrating injuries at any level, there are certain sites where the nerve is prone to injury (Sunderland, 1968). Compression neuropathies of the ulnar nerve at the elbow are common and widely recognized. In the retrocondylar groove, the nerve lies on bone covered only by a thin layer of skin and is subject to chronic compression from multiple etiologies. At 1–2 cm distally, the nerve may be entrapped at the cubital tunnel. Compression at either site may result in the clinical presentation known as *ulnar neuropathy at the elbow*. Rarely, the nerve may be entrapped in the proximal forearm as it pierces the deep aponeurosis investing the undersurface of the flexor carpi ulnaris (Amadio and Beckenbaugh, 1986; Campbell et al., 1988) or in the distal forearm by a fibrovascular band or hypertrophied flexor carpi ulnaris tendon (Campbell, 1989). Entrapment at the wrist (Guyon's canal) may present with different patterns of sensorimotor deficits, depending on the degree of involvement of the superficial (sensory) or deep (motor) branches.

ULNAR NEUROPATHY AT THE ELBOW (RETROCONDYLAR GROOVE)

Etiology

Ulnar neuropathy at the elbow can be caused by compression at the retrocondylar groove due to repeated trauma (habitual leaning on the elbows), traumatic joint deformity, distal humerus fractures, elbow dislocations, recurrent subluxation of the nerve, callus formation, rheumatic and degenerative joint disease, congenital anomalies of the medial epicondyle, epicondylo-olecranon ligament, valgus deformity, and immobilization during surgery.

General Comments

Originally, the term *tardy ulnar palsy* referred to antecedent traumatic joint deformity or recurrent subluxation. Many clinicians now use the term for any entrapment of the ulnar nerve at the elbow.

The appearance of ulnar mononeuropathy may herald the onset of a more generalized neuropathy.

Ulnar neuropathy at the retrocondylar groove should be distinguished electrodiagnostically from cubital tunnel syndrome. The distinction can be important in surgical management; the former generally requires surgical transposition of the nerve, whereas the latter may warrant simple decompression of the nerve in the tunnel, without transposition (Miller, 1991).

Clinical Features

Paresthesia, pain, or numbness occurs in the sensory distribution of the ulnar nerve, including the dorsum of the hand.

There is pain or tenderness at the elbow.

Weakness and wasting of the first dorsal interosseous and other ulnar-innervated hand muscles may occur in severe cases. Clinical evidence of weakness may preferentially involve the first dorsal interosseous (Stewart, 1987).

Weakness of the flexor carpi ulnaris and flexor digitorum profundus (to digits 4 and 5) may be variable.

Radiographic studies may visualize rheumatic, arthritic, or post-traumatic changes around the elbow.

Electrodiagnostic Strategy

Use special nerve conduction studies ("inching technique") to precisely localize the conduction abnormality (focal slowing, conduction block) to the retrocondylar region.

Use routine nerve conduction studies to demonstrate an absent or reduced ulnar dorsal cutaneous response.

Demonstrate neurogenic EMG abnormalities in the first dorsal interosseous and other ulnar-innervated hand muscles.

EMG abnormalities in the flexor carpi ulnaris and flexor digitorum profundus (superficial head) localize the lesion to the elbow. In many patients, however, these muscles may be normal, however particularly in mild ulnar neuropathy (Kincaid, 1988; Campbell et al., 1989).

ULNAR NEUROPATHY AT THE ELBOW (CUBITAL TUNNEL SYNDROME)

Etiology

Entrapment of the ulnar nerve occurs in the tunnel formed by the tendinous arch connecting the humeral and ulnar heads of the flexor carpi ulnaris 1–2 cm distal to the medial epicondyle.

General Comments

The cubital tunnel narrows when the elbow is flexed, this is important in the development of this compression neuropathy.

There is no joint deformity or prior trauma to the elbow.

Bilateral ulnar neuropathy occurs frequently.

Ulnar neuropathy at the retrocondylar groove should be distinguished electrodiagnostically from cubital tunnel syndrome. The former generally requires surgical transposition of the nerve, whereas the latter may warrant simple decompression in the tunnel, without transposition (Miller, 1991).

Clinical Features

Paresthesia, pain, or numbness occurs in the sensory distribution of the ulnar nerve, including the dorsum of the hand.

There is pain or tenderness at or slightly distal to the elbow.

In severe cases, weakness and wasting of the first dorsal interosseous and other ulnar-innervated hand muscles may occur. Clinical evidence of weakness may preferentially involve the first dorsal interosseous (Stewart, 1987).

Weakness of the flexor carpi ulnaris and flexor digitorum profundus (to digits 4 and 5) may be variable.

Radiographic studies are normal.

Electrodiagnostic Strategy

Use special nerve conduction studies ("inching technique") to precisely localize the conduction abnormality (focal slowing, conduction block) to the cubital tunnel.

Use routine nerve conduction studies to demonstrate an absent or reduced ulnar dorsal cutaneous response.

Demonstrate neurogenic EMG abnormalities in the first dorsal interosseous and other ulnar-innervated hand muscles.

EMG abnormalities in the flexor carpi ulnaris and flexor digitorum profundus (superficial head) localize the lesion to the elbow. These muscles may be normal, however, particularly in mild ulnar neuropathy (Kincaid, 1988; Campbell et al., 1989).

ULNAR NEUROPATHY AT THE WRIST (GUYON'S CANAL)

Etiology

Entrapment of the ulnar nerve occurs in the tunnel formed by the pisiform bone medially and the hook of the hamate laterally. The firm floor consists of the thick transverse carpal ligament and subjacent bone. The distal roof is rigidly bound by the piso-hamate ligament.

Entrapment may be associated with a lipoma, ganglion cyst, aneurysm, other mass lesion, or chronic compression to the hypothenar region (bicycle bars, crutches, occupation).

General Comments

Within the canal, the nerve divides into superficial (sensory) and deep (muscular) branches.

Clinical Features

Nerve or branch lesions at four different locations within Guyon's canal produce distinctive patterns of symptoms and signs (Olney and Hanson, 1988). *Pattern 1:* A deep branch lesion distal to the hypothenar motor branch produces weakness in the interossei and lumbricals but not the hypothenar muscles; there are no sensory deficits. *Pattern 2:* A lesion at or proximal to hypothenar motor branch produces weakness in the interossei, lumbricals, and hypothenar muscles; there are no sensory deficits. *Pattern 3:* A lesion at or proximal to the bifurcation into deep and superficial branches produces weakness in the interossei, lumbricals, and hypothenar muscles and sensory deficits in the distal palm, fifth digit, and ulnar side of the fourth digit. *Pattern 4:* A lesion limited to the superficial branch produces only sensory deficits in the distal palm, fifth digit, and ulnar side of the fourth digit.

Lesions that compress the deep motor branch (patterns 1 and 2) are the most common and may be confused with focal onset of amyotrophic lateral sclerosis, particularly in the all-ulnar hand.

Lesions that compress the superficial branch (patterns 3 and 4) do not produce loss of sensation over the ulnar dorsal surface of the hand (ulnar dorsal cutaneous distribution).

Electrodiagnostic Strategy

Use nerve conduction studies to localize the conduction abnormality (prolonged distal latencies in motor or sensory responses, reduced amplitudes) to the wrist. Motor conduction studies should record over the first dorsal interosseous as well as hypothenar muscles. This allows detection of distal deep branch lesions.

Elicit normal sensory nerve conduction studies of the ulnar dorsal cutaneous branch.

Demonstrate neurogenic EMG abnormalities in the first dorsal interosseous and other ulnar-innervated hand muscles.

Perform EMG in additional muscles to exclude anterior horn cell disease and C_8, T_1 radiculopathy.

REFERENCES

Amadio P C, Beckenbaugh R D: Entrapment of the ulnar nerve by the deep flexorpronator aponeurosis. J Hand Surg 1986; 11A:83–87.

Campbell W W: AAEE case report #18: Entrapment neuropathy in the distal forearm. Muscle Nerve 1989; 12:347–352.

Campbell W W, Pridgeon R M, Ria G, Crostic E G, et al: Sparing of the flexor carpi ulnaris in ulnar neuropathy at the elbow. Muscle Nerve 1989;12:965–967.

Campbell W W, Pridgeon R M, Sahni K S: Entrapment neuropathy of the ulnar nerve at its point of exit from the flexor carpi ulnaris muscle. Muscle Nerve 1988; 11:467–470.

Gray's Anatomy. 38th Edition, Churchill Livingstone, New York, 1995, pp 1266–1274.

Kincaid J C: AAEE minimonograph #31: The electrodiagnosis of ulnar neuropathy at the elbow. Muscle Nerve 1988;11:1005–1015.

Miller R G: AAEM case report #1: Ulnar neuropathy at the elbow. Muscle Nerve 1991;14: 97–101.

Olney R K, Hanson M: AAEE case report #15: Ulnar neuropathy at or distal to the wrist. Muscle Nerve 1988;11:828–832.

Stewart J D: The variable clinical manifestations of ulnar neuropathies at the elbow. J Neurol Neurosurg Psychiatry 1987;50:252–258.

Sunderland S: Nerves and Nerve Injuries. Williams & Wilkins, Baltimore, 1968, pp 808–885.

Adductor Pollicis

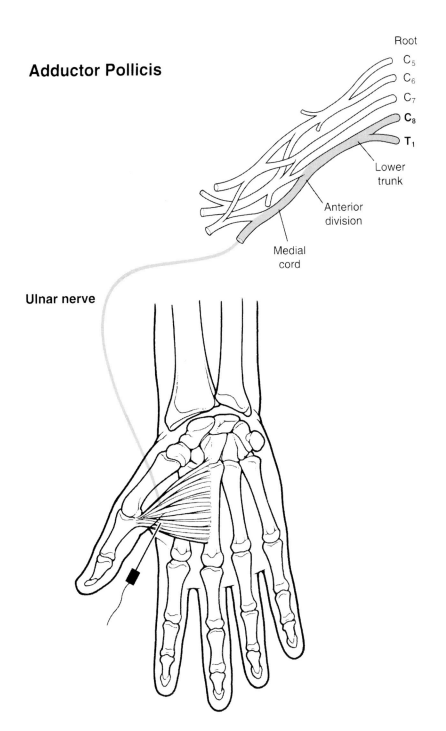

Ulnar nerve

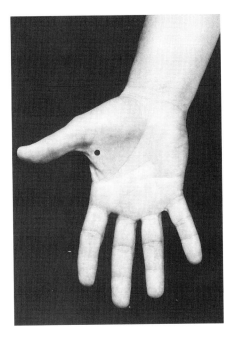

terosseous, which is also supplied by the ulnar nerve.

If the needle is inserted too anteriorly (volarly) and proximally, it may be in thenar muscles innervated by the median nerve.

Clinical Comments

This is the most distal muscle innervated by the ulnar nerve.

If ulnar-innervated muscles are atrophied, the needle is more likely to enter median-innervated thenar muscles.

In ulnar neuropathy at the wrist (Guyon's canal) or elbow (cubital tunnel, retrocondylar groove), the needle examination may show neurogenic changes when compression produces axonal loss (i.e., in moderate to severe entrapment).

In C_8, T_1 radiculopathy, the needle examination may show neurogenic changes when root pathology produces axonal loss (i.e., in moderate to severe radiculopathy).

In Klumpke's palsy (C_8, T_1 root avulsion), needle examination will show neurogenic changes.

Innervation

Innervation is via the ulnar nerve, medial cord, lower trunk, and roots C_8, T_1.

Origin

Oblique fibers arise from the capitate bone and bases of the second and third metacarpal bones; transverse fibers arise from the distal two-thirds of the metacarpal bone of the middle finger.

Insertion

Insertion is at the medial side of the base of the proximal phalanx of the thumb.

Activation Maneuver

Adduction of the thumb activates the adductor pollicis.

EMG Needle Insertion

Insert the needle into the first web space just anterior (volar) to the edge of the first dorsal interosseous and proximal to the first metacarpophalangeal joint.

Pitfalls

If the needle is inserted too posteriorly (dorsally), it will be in the first dorsal in-

Flexor Pollicis Brevis

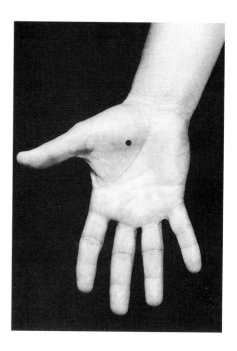

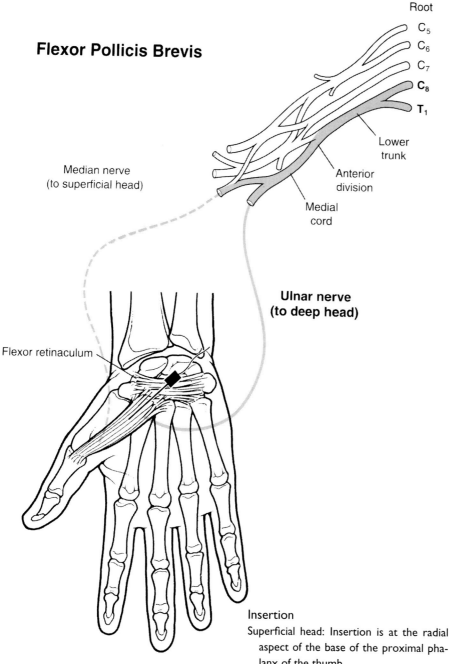

Root
C₅
C₆
C₇
C₈
T₁
Lower trunk
Anterior division
Medial cord

Median nerve (to superficial head)

Ulnar nerve (to deep head)

Flexor retinaculum

Innervation
Superficial head: Innervation is via the median nerve, medial cord, lower trunk, and roots C_8, T_1.

Deep head: Innervation is via the ulnar nerve, medial cord, lower trunk, and roots C_8, T_1.

Origin
The superficial head of the flexor pollicis brevis originates in the flexor retinaculum and trapezium.

The deep head of the flexor pollicis brevis originates in the ulnar aspect of the first metacarpal.

Insertion
Superficial head: Insertion is at the radial aspect of the base of the proximal phalanx of the thumb.

Deep head: Insertion is at the ulnar aspect of the base of the proximal phalanx of the thumb.

Activation Maneuver
Flexion of the metacarpophalangeal joint of the thumb activates the muscle.

EMG Needle Insertion
Superficial head: Insert the needle obliquely to a depth of 0.5–1 cm at the midpoint of a line drawn between the metacarpophalangeal joint and the pisiform. Assess abnormal EMG activity by directing the needle distally along the muscle.

Deep head: The procedure is the same as that for the superficial head except that the needle is inserted to a depth of 1–2 cm.

Pitfalls
If the needle is inserted too deeply, it may penetrate the opponens pollicis, which is innervated by the median nerve; if it is inserted even deeper, it may penetrate the adductor pollicis, which receives innervation from the ulnar nerve.

If the needle is inserted too laterally, it will be in the abductor pollicis brevis, which receives innervation from the median nerve.

Clinical Comments
Examination of the flexor pollicis brevis is rarely of benefit in a routine EMG needle evaluation (in general, muscles that receive dual innervation should be avoided).

The superficial head will show neurogenic changes in lesions of the median nerve.

The deep head will show neurogenic changes in lesions of the ulnar nerve.

In C_8, T_1 radiculopathy, needle examination will show neurogenic changes if root pathology has resulted in axonal loss in motor fibers (i.e., in moderate to severe radiculopathy).

In Klumpke's palsy (C_8, T_1 root avulsion), needle examination will show neurogenic changes.

First Dorsal Interosseous

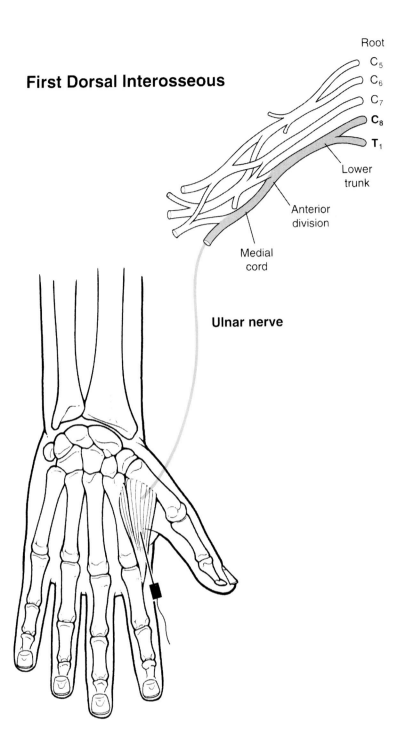

Root
C₅
C₆
C₇
C₈
T₁

Lower trunk

Anterior division

Medial cord

Ulnar nerve

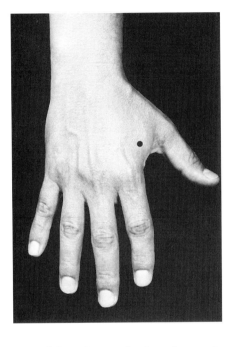

and direct it rostrally along the muscle belly.

Pitfalls
There are no pitfalls. If the needle is inserted too deeply, it will still be in C_8, T_1 muscles innervated by the ulnar nerve.

Clinical Comments
In ulnar neuropathy at the wrist (Guyon's canal), needle examination may show neurogenic changes when compression produces axonal loss (i.e., in moderate to severe entrapment).

In ulnar neuropathy at the elbow (cubital tunnel, retrocondylar groove), needle examination may show neurogenic changes when compression produces axonal loss.

In C_8, T_1 radiculopathy, needle examination may show neurogenic changes when root pathology produces axonal loss (i.e., in moderate to severe radiculopathy).

In Klumpke's palsy (C_8, T_1 root avulsion), needle examination will show neurogenic changes.

Innervation
Innervation is via the ulnar nerve, medial cord, lower trunk, and roots C_8, T_1.

Origin
The first dorsal interosseous originates at the ulnar border of the first metacarpal bone (outer head) and the radial border of the second metacarpal bone (inner head).

Insertion
Insertion is at the radial aspect of the base of the proximal phalanx of the index finger.

Activation Maneuver
Abduction (radial deviation) of the index finger activates the muscle.

EMG Needle Insertion
Insert the needle obliquely just proximal to the second metacarpophalangeal joint,

2nd, 3rd, 4th Dorsal Interossei

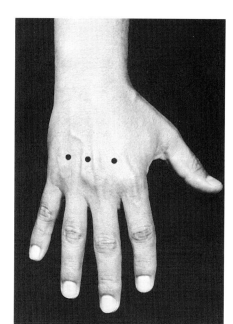

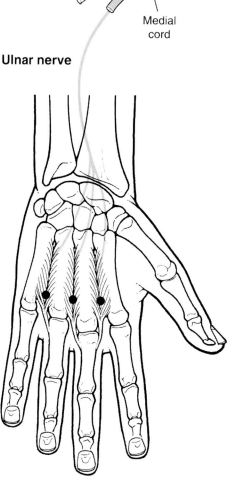

Root
C₅
C₆
C₇
C₈
T₁

Lower trunk

Anterior division

Medial cord

Ulnar nerve

Activation Maneuver

Second: Abduction (radial deviation) of the third digit activates the muscle.

Third and fourth: Adduction (ulnar deviation) of the third and fourth digit, respectively, activates the muscle.

EMG Needle Insertion

Second: Insert the needle just radial to the third metacarpal bone.

Third and fourth: Insert the needle just ulnar to the third and fourth metacarpal bones, respectively.

Pitfalls

There are no pitfalls. If the needle is inserted too deeply, it will still be in C_8, T_1 muscles innervated by the ulnar nerve.

Clinical Comments

The interossei are occasionally doubled in one or more spaces, or they may be absent in one or more spaces.

There may be variable innervation to these muscles from the median nerve.

Examination of the interossei causes pain and is rarely of benefit in a routine EMG needle evaluation.

In ulnar neuropathy at the wrist (Guyon's canal), needle examination may show neurogenic changes when compression produces axonal loss (i.e., in moderate to severe entrapment).

In ulnar neuropathy at the elbow (cubital tunnel, retrocondylar groove), needle examination may show neurogenic changes when compression produces axonal loss.

In C_8, T_1 radiculopathy, needle examination may show neurogenic changes when root pathology produces axonal loss (i.e., in moderate to severe radiculopathy).

In Klumpke's palsy (C_8, T_1 root avulsion), needle examination will show neurogenic changes.

Innervation

Innervation is via the ulnar nerve, medial cord, lower trunk, and roots C_8, T_1.

Origin

The second dorsal interosseous originates at the radial border of the third metacarpal bone and the ulnar border of the second metacarpal bone.

The third and fourth dorsal interossei originate at the ulnar border of the third and fourth metacarpal bones and the radial border of the fourth and fifth metacarpal bones, respectively.

Insertion

Second: Insertion is at the radial aspect of the base of the proximal phalanx of the third digit.

Third and fourth: Insertion is at the ulnar aspect of the base of the proximal phalanx of the third and fourth digit, respectively.

Palmar Interossei

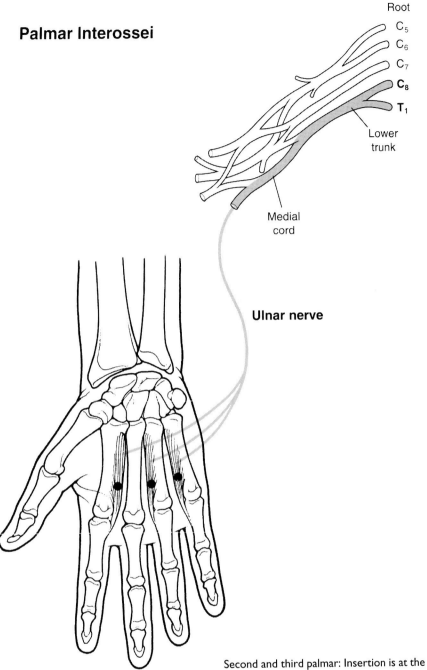

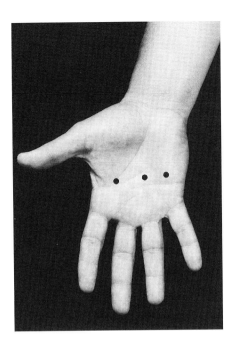

Innervation
Innervation is via the ulnar nerve, medial cord, lower trunk, and roots C_8, T_1.

Origin
The first palmar interosseous originates at ulnar aspect of the second metacarpal bone.

The second and third palmar interossei originate at the radial aspect of the fourth and fifth metacarpal bones, respectively.

Insertion
First palmar: Insertion is at the ulnar side of the proximal phalanx of the second digit.

Second and third palmar: Insertion is at the radial side of the proximal phalanges of the fourth and fifth digits, respectively.

Activation Maneuver
The palmar interossei adduct the fingers to an imaginary line drawn longitudinally through the center of the third digit (middle finger). The first palmar performs ulnar deviation of the second digit; the second and third palmars perform radial deviation of the fourth and fifth digits, respectively.

EMG Needle Insertion
First palmar: Insert the needle just ulnar to the second metacarpal bone.

Second and third palmars: Insert the needle just radial to the fourth and fifth metacarpal bones, respectively.

Pitfalls
There are no pitfalls. If the needle is inserted too deeply, it will still be in C_8, T_1 muscles innervated by the ulnar nerve.

Clinical Comments
The interossei are occasionally doubled in one or more spaces, or they may be absent in one or more spaces.

There may be variable innervation to these muscles from the median nerve.

Examination of the palmar interossei causes pain and is rarely of benefit in a routine EMG needle evaluation.

In ulnar neuropathy at the wrist (Guyon's canal), needle examination may show neurogenic changes when compression produces axonal loss (i.e., in moderate to severe entrapment).

In ulnar neuropathy at the elbow (cubital tunnel, retrocondylar groove), needle examination may show neurogenic changes when compression produces axonal loss.

In C_8, T_1 radiculopathy, needle examination may show neurogenic changes when root pathology produces axonal loss (i.e., in moderate to severe radiculopathy).

In Klumpke's palsy (C_8, T_1 root avulsion), needle examination will show neurogenic changes.

3rd, 4th Lumbricals

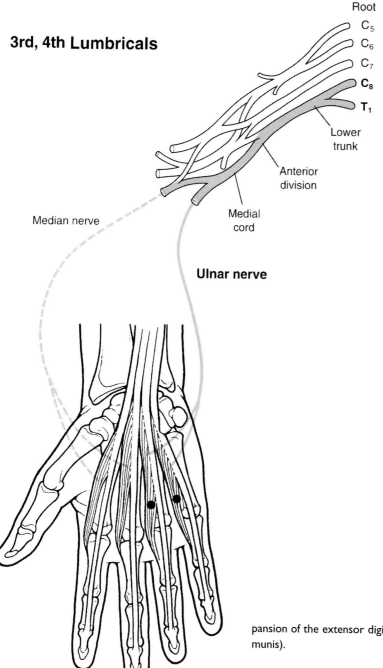

Root
C₅
C₆
C₇
C₈
T₁

Lower trunk

Anterior division

Median nerve

Medial cord

Ulnar nerve

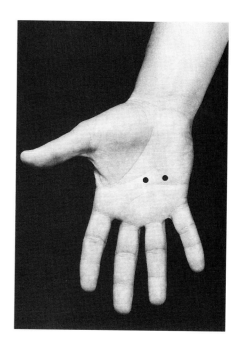

Innervation
Innervation is via the ulnar nerve, medial cord, lower trunk, and roots C₈, T₁.

Origin
The third and fourth lumbricals originate at the radial aspect of the tendon sheath of the flexor digitorum profundus.

Insertion
Insertion is at the radial lateral band of the dorsal digital expansion (tendinous ex-

pansion of the extensor digitorum communis).

Activation Maneuver
Extension of the finger at the proximal interphalangeal joint with the metacarpophalangeal joint extended and fixed activates the muscles.

EMG Needle Insertion
Insert the needle just proximal to the metacarpophalangeal joint and radial to the flexor tendon.

Pitfalls
There are no pitfalls. All muscles surrounding the third and fourth lumbricals receive innervation from the ulnar nerve.

Clinical Comments
Examination of the third and fourth lumbricals causes pain and is rarely of benefit in a routine EMG needle evaluation.

In ulnar neuropathy at the wrist (Guyon's canal), needle examination may show neurogenic changes when compression produces axonal loss (i.e., in moderate to severe entrapment.

In ulnar neuropathy at the elbow (cubital tunnel, retrocondylar groove), needle examination may show neurogenic changes when compression produces axonal loss.

In C₈, T₁ radiculopathy, needle examination may show neurogenic changes when root pathology produces axonal loss (i.e., in moderate to severe radiculopathy).

In Klumpke's palsy (C₈, T₁ root avulsion), needle examination will show neurogenic changes.

Abductor Digiti Minimi

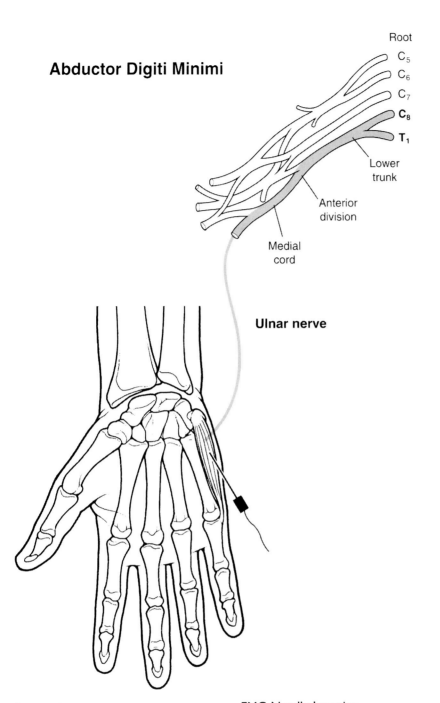

Root
C₅
C₆
C₇
C₈
T₁

Lower trunk

Anterior division

Medial cord

Ulnar nerve

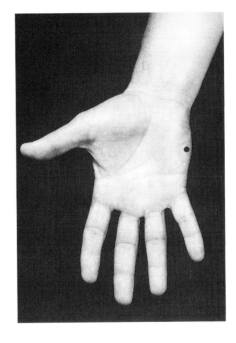

Innervation
Innervation is via the ulnar nerve, medial cord, lower trunk, and roots C_8, T_1.

Origin
The abductor digit minimi originate at the pisiform bone.

Insertion
Insertion is at the medial side of the base of the proximal phalanx of the little finger.

Activation Maneuver
Abduction of the little finger activates the muscles.

EMG Needle Insertion
Insert the needle obliquely at the midpoint between the fifth metacarpophalangeal joint (metacarpophalangeal crease) and the ulnar aspect of the pisiform (distal wrist crease).

Pitfalls
There are no pitfalls. If the needle is inserted too deeply or laterally, it will still be in C_8, T_1 muscles innervated by the ulnar nerve.

Clinical Comments
In ulnar neuropathy at the wrist (Guyon's canal), needle examination may show neurogenic changes when compression produces axonal loss (i.e., in moderate to severe entrapment).

In ulnar neuropathy at the elbow (cubital tunnel, retrocondylar groove), needle examination may show neurogenic changes when compression produces axonal loss.

In C_8, T_1 radiculopathy, needle examination may show neurogenic changes when root pathology produces axonal loss (i.e., in moderate to severe radiculopathy).

In Klumpke's palsy (C_8, T_1 root avulsion), needle examination will show neurogenic changes.

Opponens Digiti Minimi

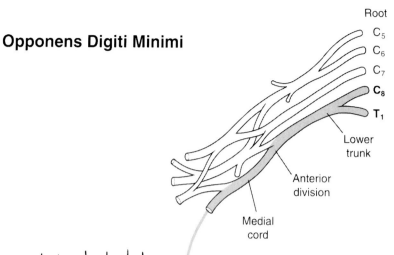

Root
C₅
C₆
C₇
C₈
T₁
Lower trunk
Anterior division
Medial cord

Ulnar nerve

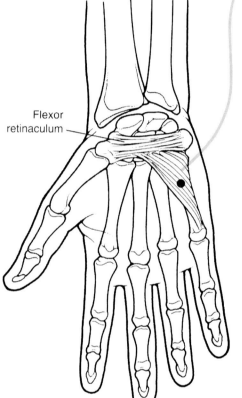

Flexor retinaculum

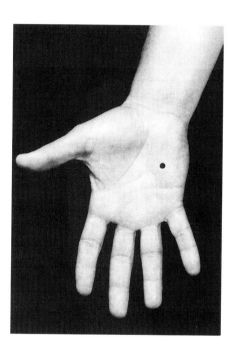

Innervation
Innervation is via the ulnar nerve, medial cord, lower trunk, and roots C₈, T₁.

Origin
The opponens digiti minimi originate at the flexor retinaculum and the hook of the hamate.

Insertion
Insertion is at the ulnar margin of the fifth metacarpal bone.

Activation Maneuver
Opposition of the little finger to the thumb activates the muscles.

EMG Needle Insertion
Insert the needle at the midpoint between the fifth metacarpophalangeal joint (metacarpophalangeal crease) and the pisiform (distal wrist crease), just radial to the abductor digiti minimi.

Pitfalls
There are no pitfalls. If the needle is inserted too deeply or laterally, it will still be in C₈, T₁ muscles innervated by the ulnar nerve.

Clinical Comments
In ulnar neuropathy at the wrist (Guyon's canal), needle examination may show neurogenic changes when compression produces axonal loss (i.e., in moderate to severe entrapment).

In ulnar neuropathy at the elbow (cubital tunnel, retrocondylar groove), needle examination may show neurogenic changes when compression produces axonal loss.

In C₈, T₁ radiculopathy, needle examination may show neurogenic changes when root pathology produces axonal loss (i.e., in moderate to severe radiculopathy).

In Klumpke's palsy (C₈, T₁ root avulsion), needle examination will show neurogenic changes.

Flexor Digiti Minimi

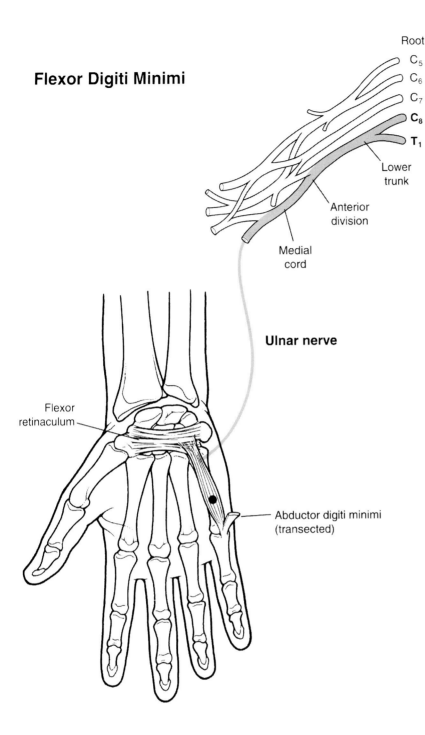

Root
C₅
C₆
C₇
C₈
T₁

Lower trunk

Anterior division

Medial cord

Ulnar nerve

Flexor retinaculum

Abductor digiti minimi (transected)

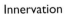

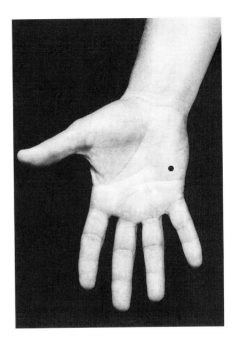

Innervation
Innervation is via the ulnar nerve, medial cord, lower trunk, and roots C₈, T₁.

Origin
The flexor digiti minimi originate at the hook of the hamate and the flexor retinaculum.

Insertion
Insertion is at the ulnar side of the base of the proximal phalanx of the little finger.

Activation Maneuver
Flexion of the proximal phalanx of the fifth digit activates the muscles.

EMG Needle Insertion
Insert the needle at the midpoint between the fifth metacarpophalangeal joint (metacarpophalangeal crease) and the ulnar aspect of the pisiform (distal wrist crease), just radial to the abductor digiti minimi.

Pitfalls
There are no pitfalls. If the needle is inserted too deeply, it will be in the opponens digiti minimi, which is still innervated by the ulnar nerve.

Clinical Comments
In ulnar neuropathy at the wrist (Guyon's canal), needle examination may show neurogenic changes when compression produces axonal loss (i.e., in moderate to severe entrapment).

In ulnar neuropathy at the elbow (cubital tunnel, retrocondylar groove), needle examination may show neurogenic changes when compression produces axonal loss.

In C₈, T₁ radiculopathy, needle examination may show neurogenic changes when root pathology produces axonal loss (i.e., in moderate to severe radiculopathy).

In Klumpke's palsy (C₈, T₁ root avulsion), needle examination will show neurogenic changes.

Flexor Digitorum Profundus
Digits 4 and 5

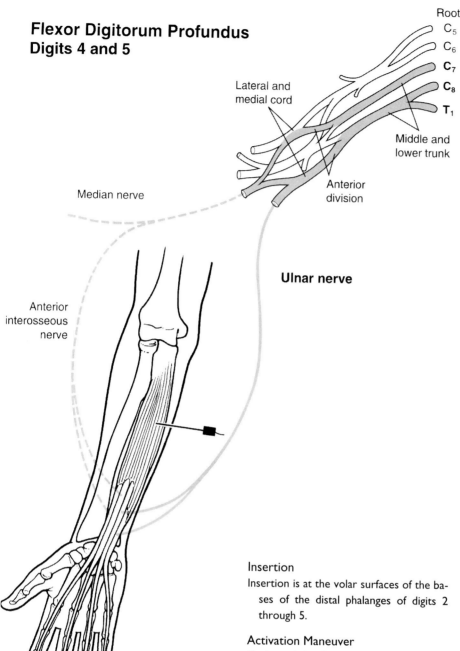

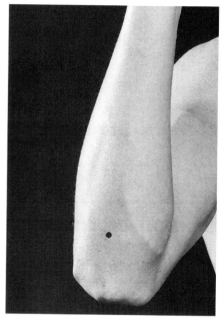

Innervation
Digits four and five: Innervation is via the ulnar nerve, medial cord, lower trunk, and roots C8, T1.

Digits two and three: Innervation is via the anterior interosseous branch, median nerve, lateral and medial cords, middle and lower trunks, and roots C7, C8.

Origin
The flexor digitorum profundus originates at the volar and medial surfaces of the shaft of the ulna.

Insertion
Insertion is at the volar surfaces of the bases of the distal phalanges of digits 2 through 5.

Activation Maneuver
Flexion of the distal phalanges of digits 4 and 5 activates the muscle.

EMG Needle Insertion
Palpate the shaft of the ulna along the medial forearm. Insert the needle 5–7 cm distal to the olecranon process and 1–1.5 cm medial to the shaft of the ulna. The ulna-innervated portion lies superficially at a depth of 1–2 cm; the median portion lies deep at a depth of 3–4 cm. Note: The easiest approach to this muscle is for the subject to place the forearm perpendicular to the table with the hand and wrist relaxed. The shaft of the ulna and the adjacent belly of the muscle can easily be palpated (see photograph).

Pitfalls
If the needle is inserted too volary (i.e., toward the palmar surface), it may lie in the flexor carpi ulnaris, which also receives innervation from the ulnar nerve.

Clinical Comments
Needle examination of the superficial portion may show neurogenic changes in axonal loss lesions of the ulnar nerve at the elbow (cubital tunnel or retrocondylar groove).

Needle examination of the deep portion may show neurogenic changes if a lesion of the anterior interosseous nerve produces axonal loss and in axonal loss lesions of the median nerve at the elbow (pronator teres syndrome) or above the elbow (ligament of Struther's syndrome).

In C8, T1 radiculopathy, the needle examination may show neurogenic changes when root pathology has resulted in axonal loss (i.e., in moderate to severe radiculopathy).

In Klumpke's palsy (C8, T1 root avulsion), needle examination will show neurogenic changes.

Flexor Carpi Ulnaris

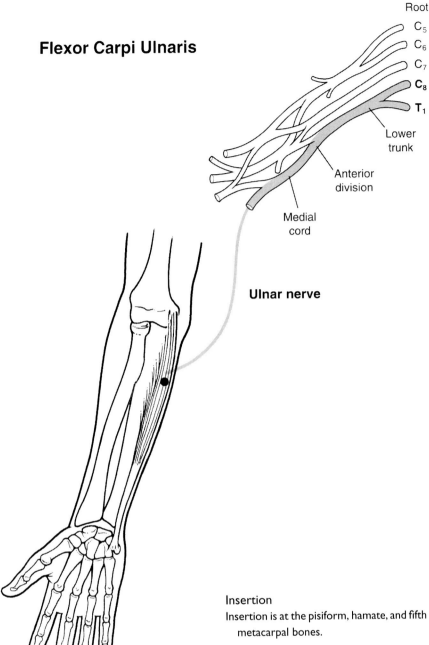

Root
C₅
C₆
C₇
C₈
T₁
Lower trunk
Anterior division
Medial cord

Ulnar nerve

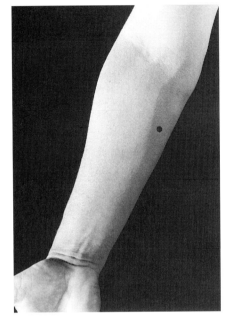

Innervation
Innervation is via the ulnar nerve, medial cord, lower trunk, and roots C_8, T_1.

Origin
The flexor carpi ulnaris arises by two heads. One head is from the medial epicondyle of the humerus, and the other head is from the olecranon process and the upper two-thirds of the posterior border of the ulna.

Insertion
Insertion is at the pisiform, hamate, and fifth metacarpal bones.

Activation Maneuver
Flexion at the wrist with ulnar deviation activates the muscles.

EMG Needle Insertion
Insert the needle 5–8 cm distal to the medial epicondyle along a line connecting the medial epicondyle and pisiform bone.

Pitfalls
If the needle is inserted too laterally (radially), it may be in the palmaris longus or the flexor carpi radialis, both muscles innervated by the median nerve.

If the needle is inserted too deeply, it may be in the flexor digitorum superficialis (supplied by median nerve), or, if still deeper, it may penetrate the flexor digitorum profundus (supplied by median and ulnar nerves).

Clinical Comments
The two heads are connected by a tendinous arch that forms the cubital tunnel 1–2 cm distal to the medial epicondyle, through which passes the ulnar nerve. Entrapment at this site produces ulnar neuropathy at the elbow (cubital tunnel).

Needle examination of this muscle is usually normal in cubital tunnel entrapment. It may also be normal in ulnar neuropathy due to compression at the retrocondylar groove.

In C_8, T_1 radiculopathy, needle examination may show neurogenic changes when root pathology produces axonal loss (i.e., in moderate to severe radiculopathy).

In Klumpke's palsy (C_8, T_1 root avulsion), needle examination will show neurogenic changes.

chapter

4

Radial

Nerve

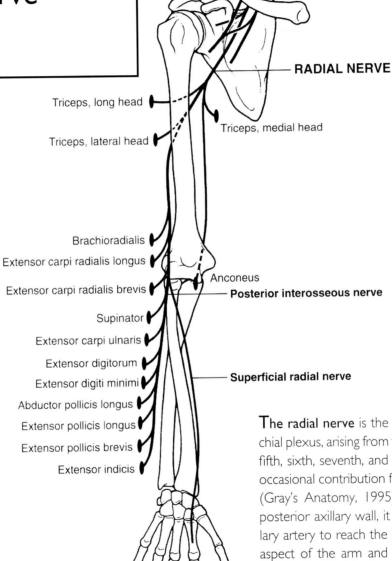

RADIAL NERVE

Triceps, long head

Triceps, lateral head

Triceps, medial head

Brachioradialis
Extensor carpi radialis longus
Extensor carpi radialis brevis

Anconeus
Posterior interosseous nerve

Supinator
Extensor carpi ulnaris
Extensor digitorum
Extensor digiti minimi

Superficial radial nerve

Abductor pollicis longus
Extensor pollicis longus
Extensor pollicis brevis
Extensor indicis

Diagram of the radial nerve and the muscles that it supplies.

The radial nerve is the largest branch of the brachial plexus, arising from the posterior cord and the fifth, sixth, seventh, and eighth cervical roots, with occasional contribution from the first thoracic root (Gray's Anatomy, 1995). From its origin on the posterior axillary wall, it descends behind the axillary artery to reach the angle between the medial aspect of the arm and the posterior wall of the axilla (brachio-axillary angle). Branches to the heads of the triceps and anconeus arise in the axilla and brachio-axillary angle.

With the profunda brachii artery, the radial nerve inclines downward between the long and medial heads of the triceps, after which it passes obliquely along the back of the humerus in the spiral groove (also known as the *radial groove*). Here it is in direct contact with bone. On reaching the lateral side of the humerus, the nerve pierces the lateral intermuscular septum to enter the anterior compartment. It then descends in the furrow between the brachialis medially and brachioradialis laterally. The nerve gives off branches to the brachialis (this muscle is supplied primarily by the musculocutaneous nerve) and brachioradialis. The nerve is overlapped, in turn, by the extensor carpi radialis longus and extensor carpi radialis brevis. The radial nerve supplies both muscles, although the extensor carpi radialis brevis may receive its nerve supply from the superficial radial or posterior interosseous nerve (Sunderland, 1968).

Anterior to the lateral epicondyle, the radial nerve divides into its two terminal branches: the posterior interosseous nerve and the superficial radial nerve. The former is a pure muscular nerve that innervates the supinator before passing through the arcade formed by the superficial and deep heads of this muscle (arcade of Frohse). On the dorsum of the forearm, the posterior interosseous nerve divides in a variable manner to innervate the extensor carpi ulnaris, extensor digitorum communis, extensor digiti minimi, abductor pollicis longus, extensor pollicis longus and brevis, and extensor indicis. The superficial radial branch is primarily a sensory nerve. It provides cutaneous innervation to the dorsum of the hand lateral to the ring finger, dorsum of the thumb, radial aspect of the thenar eminence, and dorsum of the index, middle, and radial half of the ring fingers as far distally as the middle phalanx.

Although the radial nerve, or its branches, may be involved in penetrating injuries at any level, there are certain sites where the nerve is more prone to injury (Sunderland, 1968). In the brachio-axillary angle, compression may result from a misused crutch or from fractures of the upper third of the humerus. In the region of the spiral groove and lateral intermuscular septum, compression neuropathies of the radial nerve are common and widely recognized. The nerve is most commonly damaged by fractures of the humerus or during deep intoxication with the arm draped over the edge of a bed, chair, or bench (Saturday night palsy). In its course through the supinator (arcade of Frohse), the posterior interosseous nerve is prone to damage from fractures of the upper third of the radius and less commonly from entrapment. Injury to the superficial radial branch may result from tight handcuffs (handcuff neuropathy) or carelessly administered intravenous infusions.

RADIAL NERVE LESION IN THE ARM

Etiology

Compression of the nerve in the spiral groove (radial groove) of the humerus can cause a radial nerve lesion in the arm.

The condition is called "Saturday night palsy" when sedatives or alcohol produces deep sleep in someone and an arm is draped over the edge of a bed, chair, or bench.

The condition is called "honeymooner's palsy" when compression results from the weight of a partner's head lying on the arm.

A radial nerve lesion can occur secondary to a fracture of the humerus, prolonged or excessive muscle contraction (as in masons, carpenters, or athletes in throwing sports), anatomical anomalies of the triceps, and deep intramuscular injections.

General Comments

A radial nerve lesion in the arm is a common compression neuropathy.

Predisposing factors include diabetes, malnutrition, alcohol or sedative use, and hereditary susceptibility to pressure palsies (Brown and Watson, 1993).

The differential diagnosis includes lead poisoning, porphyria, diabetes, and periarteritis nodosa.

Clinical Features

Wrist drop occurs with a radial nerve lesion in the arm.

There is normal function of the triceps (extension of forearm at elbow).

There is weakness of the brachioradialis and all other muscles supplied by the radial nerve beyond the spiral groove.

Pain is not a typical feature, but it may be perceived in the area of the lateral epicondyle, radial styloid, or dorsum of hand.

Numbness can occur in the distribution of the superficial radial nerve and occasionally in the territory of the posterior cutaneous nerve of the forearm.

Most cases of "Saturday night palsy" fully resolve in days to a few weeks, which is consistent primarily with a demyelinating lesion. Delayed or incomplete recovery implies a greater degree of axonal loss.

Electrodiagnostic Strategy

Use electrodiagnostic evaluation to confirm a focal lesion (conduction block, slowing of conduction velocity) at the spiral groove and to obtain information on severity and prognosis. Cases characterized by conduction block resolve quickly; those with axonal loss and wallerian degeneration show a reduction of motor or sensory amplitudes and resolve slowly or incompletely.

In cases of axonal loss, EMG may show neurogenic changes (spontaneous activity, abnormal motor unit potentials, and abnormal recruitment) in the brachioradialis and in all other muscles supplied by the radial nerve distal to the spiral groove.

EMG is normal in cases of demyelination and in the early stages of axonal loss in which wallerian degeneration has not yet occurred.

EMG of the triceps is normal.

The superficial radial sensory response is reduced in amplitude or absent in cases of axonal loss (normal in cases of demyelination and in the early stages of axonal loss).

EMG of nonradial innervated C_7 muscles may be necessary to exclude C_7 radiculopathy.

RADIAL NERVE LESION IN THE AXILLA

Etiology

Compression of the nerve in the axilla by high-riding crutches can cause the
condition called *crutch neuropathy*.

A radial nerve lesion can occur secondary to shoulder trauma, humerus
fractures, tumor, or anatomical anomalies of the coracobrachialis or triceps.

Clinical Features

Wrist drop occurs with a radial nerve lesion in the axilla.

Weakness occurs in all muscles supplied by the radial nerve, including the
triceps.

The triceps reflex is absent.

Numbness occurs in the distribution of the superficial radial nerve and occasionally in the the territory of the posterior cutaneous nerve of the
forearm.

Most cases fully resolve in days to a few weeks, which is consistent primarily
with a demyelinating lesion. Delayed or incomplete recovery implies a
greater degree of axonal loss.

Electrodiagnostic Strategy

Use electrodiagnostic evaluation to obtain evaluation to obtain information
on severity and prognosis. Cases associated with axonal loss and wallerian
degeneration show a reduction of motor or sensory amplitudes and resolve slowly or incompletely.

In cases of axonal loss, EMG may show neurogenic changes in the triceps
and all other muscles supplied by the radial nerve.

EMG is normal in cases of demyelination and in the early stages of axonal
loss in which wallerian degeneration has not yet occurred.

The superficial radial sensory response is reduced in amplitude or absent in
cases of axonal loss (normal in cases of demyelination and in the early
stages of axonal loss).

EMG of nonradial innervated C_7 muscles may be necessary to exclude C_7
radiculopathy.

POSTERIOR INTEROSSEOUS NERVE SYNDROME

Etiology

Compression of the nerve as it passes between the two layers of the supinator muscle in the arcade of Frohse can cause posterior interosseous
nerve syndrome.

Posterior interosseous nerve syndrome can occur secondary to radial subluxation, a fracture of the proximal radius, prolonged or repeated pronation–supination movements, tumors (lipoma), neuralgic amyotrophy,
and compression by the extensor carpi radialis brevis.

General Comments

Posterior interosseous nerve syndrome is also known as the *supinator syndrome*.

Injury to the posterior interosseous nerve is usually associated with trauma (fractures, gunshot wounds, lacerations) rather than with true entrapment.

Clinical Features

There is normal supination of the forearm and radial wrist extension (supinator and extensor carpi radialis are normal).

Weakness occurs in the extensor carpi ulnaris; attempted wrist extension results in characteristic radial deviation of the wrist.

Weakness occurs during finger extension and thumb extension. Thumb abduction may be normal because the abductor pollicis brevis (median nerve) is unaffected.

There is pain in the lateral upper forearm (usually 5–8 cm distal to the lateral epicondyle).

There is no sensory impairment because the superficial radial nerve arises above the arcade of Frohse.

Electrodiagnostic Strategy

The superficial radial sensory response is normal.

Motor studies may reveal a focal lesion (conduction block, slowing of conduction velocity) across the entrapment (Kimura, 1989). Cases characterized by conduction block resolve quickly; those associated with wallerian degeneration show a reduction of motor amplitude and resolve slowly or incompletely.

EMG may show neurogenic changes (spontaneous activity, abnormal motor unit potentials, and abnormal recruitment) in all muscles supplied by the posterior interosseous nerve below the supinator.

EMG of radial innervated muscles (triceps, anconeus, brachioradialis, and extensor carpi radialis longus and brevis) is normal.

REFERENCES

Brown W F, Watson B V: AAEM case report #27: Acute retrohumeral radial neuropathies. Muscle Nerve 1993; 16: 706–711.

Gray's Anatomy. 38th Edition. Churchill Livingstone, New York, 1995, pp 1266–1274.

Kimura J: Electrodiagnosis in Diseases of Nerve and Muscle. 2nd Edition. FA Davis, Philadelphia, 1989, pp 499–500.

Sunderland S: Nerves and Nerve Injuries. Williams & Wilkins, Baltimore, 1968, pp 894–938.

Extensor Indicis

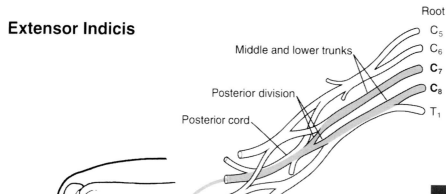

Root
C₅
C₆
C₇
C₈
T₁

Middle and lower trunks

Posterior division

Posterior cord

Radial nerve

Posterior interosseous nerve

5 to 7cm

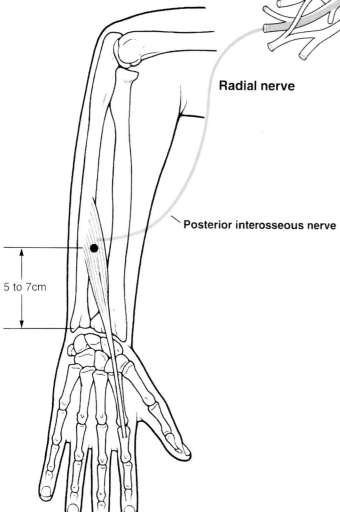

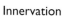

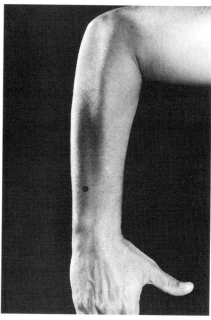

Innervation

Innervation is via the posterior interosseous nerve, radial nerve, posterior cord, middle and lower trunks, and roots C₇, C₈.

Origin

The extensor indicis originates at the posterior surface of the lower half of the shaft of the ulna and adjacent interosseous membrane.

Insertion

The extensor indicis joins the tendon of the extensor digitorum communis to the index finger.

Activation Maneuver

Extension of the index finger activates the muscle.

EMG Needle Insertion

Insert the needle 5–7 cm proximal to the ulnar styloid just radial to the shaft of the ulna. Hint: Follow the tendon proximally to where it intersects the ulna.

Pitfalls

If the needle is inserted too laterally (radially), it may be in the extensor pollicis longus, which also receives innervation from the posterior interosseous nerve.

Clinical Comments

The extensor indicis is usually the most distal muscle innervated by the posterior interosseous branch of the radial nerve.

In a radial nerve lesion at the axilla (crutch neuropathy), needle examination may show neurogenic changes when compression produces axonal loss.

In a radial nerve lesion at the upper arm (Saturday night palsy), needle examination may show neurogenic changes when compression at the spiral groove produces axonal loss.

In a posterior interosseous nerve lesion, needle examination may show neurogenic changes when pathology produces axonal loss.

Extensor Pollicis Brevis

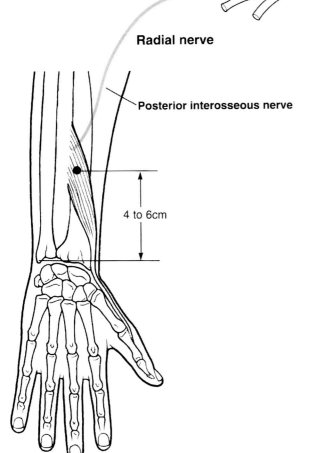

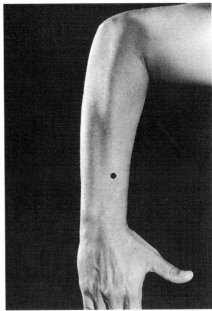

Radial nerve

Posterior interosseous nerve

4 to 6cm

Root
C₅
C₆
C₇
C₈
T₁

Middle and lower trunks

Posterior division

Posterior cord

Innervation
Innervation is via the posterior interosseous nerve, radial nerve, posterior cord, middle and lower trunks, and roots C_7, C_8.

Origin
The extensor pollicis brevis originates at the posterior surface of the shaft of the radius, below the origin of the abductor pollicis longus, and adjacent interosseous membrane.

Insertion
Insertion is at the base of the first phalanx of the thumb. (Note: The tendon passes through the same groove as the abductor pollicis longus tendon on the outer side of the styloid process, forming the radial border of the anatomical "snuffbox.")

Activation Maneuver
Extension of the proximal phalanx of the thumb activates the muscle.

EMG Needle Insertion
Insert the needle 4–6 cm proximal to the wrist over the ulnar aspect of the radius.

Pitfalls
If the needle is inserted too proximally, it may be in the abductor pollicis longus, which also receives innervation from the posterior interosseous nerve.

Clinical Comments
In a radial nerve lesion at the axilla (crutch neuropathy), needle examination may show neurogenic changes when compression produces axonal loss.

In a radial nerve lesion at the upper arm (Saturday night palsy), needle examination may show neurogenic changes when compression at the spiral groove produces axonal loss.

In a posterior interosseous nerve lesion, needle examination may show neurogenic changes when pathology produces axonal loss.

Extensor Pollicis Longus

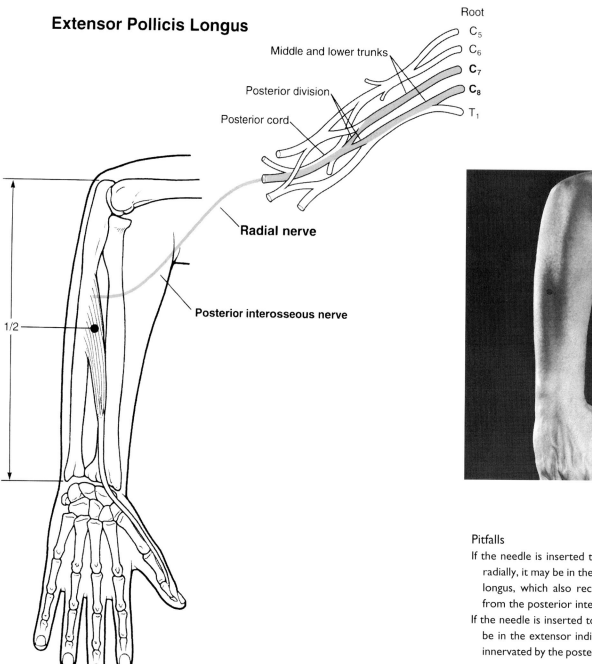

Root
- C$_5$
- C$_6$
- **C$_7$**
- **C$_8$**
- T$_1$

Middle and lower trunks

Posterior division

Posterior cord

Radial nerve

Posterior interosseous nerve

1/2

Innervation
Innervation is via the posterior interosseous nerve, radial nerve, posterior cord, middle and lower trunks, and roots C$_7$, C$_8$.

Origin
The extensor pollicis longus originates at the posterior surface of the shaft of the ulna, below the origin of the abductor pollicis longus.

Insertion
Insertion is at the base of the terminal phalanx of the thumb. (Note: The tendon forms the ulnar border of the anatomical "snuffbox.")

Activation Maneuver
Extension of the distal phalanx of the thumb activates the muscle.

EMG Needle Insertion
Insert the needle at the mid-forearm along the radial border of the ulna.

Pitfalls
If the needle is inserted too proximally or radially, it may be in the abductor pollicis longus, which also receives innervation from the posterior interosseous nerve.

If the needle is inserted too distally, it may be in the extensor indicts, which is also innervated by the posterior interosseous nerve.

Clinical Comments
In a radial nerve lesion at the axilla (crutch neuropathy), needle examination may show neurogenic changes when compression produces axonal loss.

In a radial nerve lesion at the upper arm (Saturday night palsy), needle examination may show neurogenic changes when compression at the spiral groove produces axonal loss.

In a posterior interosseous nerve lesion, needle examination may show neurogenic changes when pathology produces axonal loss.

Abductor Pollicis Longus

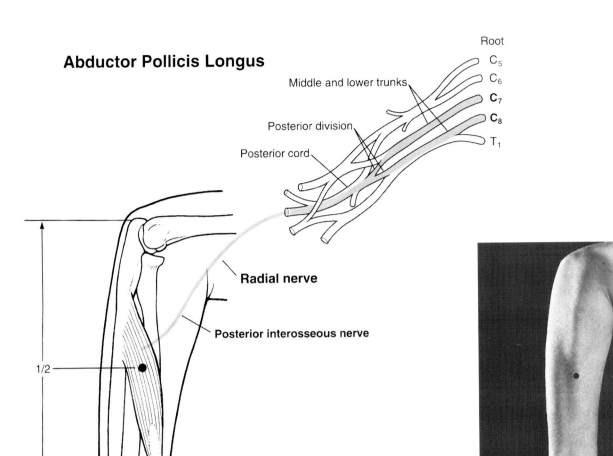

Root
C5
C6
C7
C8
T1

Middle and lower trunks

Posterior division

Posterior cord

Radial nerve

Posterior interosseous nerve

1/2

Innervation
Innervation is via the posterior interosseous nerve, radial nerve, posterior cord, middle and lower trunks, and roots C7, C8.

Origin
The abductor pollicis longus originates at the posterior surface of the shaft of the ulna, above the origin of the extensor pollicis longus; at the posterior surface of the shaft of the radius, above the origin of the extensor pollicis brevis; and at the adjacent interosseous membrane.

Insertion
Insertion is at the base of the metacarpal bone of the thumb. (Note: The tendon forms the radial border of the anatomical "snuffbox.")

Activation Maneuver
Radial abduction and extension of the thumb activate the muscle.

EMG Needle Insertion
Insert the needle at the mid-forearm along the shaft of the radius.

Pitfalls
If the needle is inserted too distally, it may be in the extensor pollicis brevis, which also receives innervation from the posterior interosseous nerve.

If the needle is inserted too proximally, it may be in the extensor carpi radialis, which is innervated by the radial nerve.

If the needle is inserted too medially (ulnarly), it may be in the extensor digitorum communis, which also receives innervation from the posterior interosseous nerve.

Clinical Comments
In a radial nerve lesion at the axilla (crutch neuropathy), needle examination may show neurogenic changes when compression produces axonal loss.

In a radial nerve lesion at the upper arm (Saturday night palsy), needle examination may show neurogenic changes when compression at the spiral groove produces axonal loss.

In a posterior interosseous nerve lesion, needle examination may show neurogenic changes when pathology produces axonal loss.

Extensor Digitorum Communis and Extensor Digiti Minimi

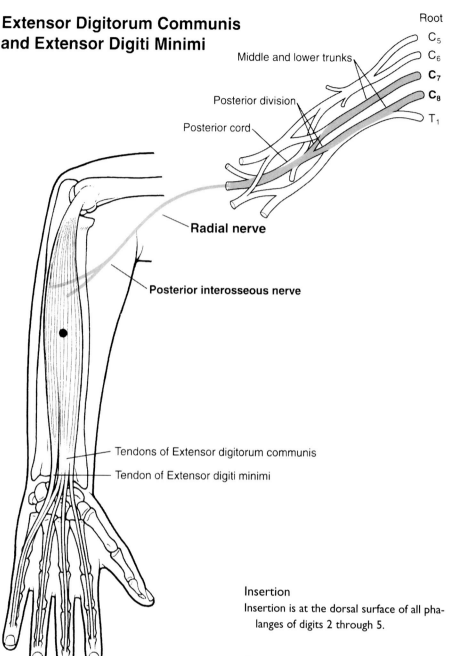

Root
C₅
C₆
C₇
C₈
T₁

Middle and lower trunks

Posterior division

Posterior cord

Radial nerve

Posterior interosseous nerve

Tendons of Extensor digitorum communis
Tendon of Extensor digiti minimi

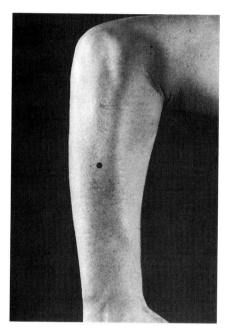

Innervation

Innervation is via the posterior interosseous nerve, radial nerve, posterior cord, middle and lower trunks, and roots C_7, C_8.

Origin

The extensor digitorum communis and extensor digiti minimi originate at the common extensor tendon from the lateral epicondyle of the humerus.

Insertion

Insertion is at the dorsal surface of all phalanges of digits 2 through 5.

Activation Maneuver

Extension of the phalanges in digits 2 through 5 activates the muscles. (Note: These muscles act principally on the proximal phalanges, the middle and distal phalanges being extended by the lumbricals and interossei.)

EMG Needle Insertion

Insert the needle in the mid-forearm midway between the ulna and radius. The extensor digiti minimi is frequently fused with the extensor digitorum communis. The extensor digiti minimi can be found in the mid-forearm on the ulnar border of the extensor digitorum communis.

Pitfalls

If the needle is inserted too laterally (radially), it may be in the extensor carpi radialis, which is innervated by the radial nerve.

If the needle is inserted too medially (ulnarly), it may be in the extensor carpi ulnaris, which also receives innervation from the posterior interosseous nerve.

Clinical Comments

In a radial nerve lesion at the axilla (crutch neuropathy), needle examination may show neurogenic changes when compression produces axonal loss.

In a radial nerve lesion at the upper arm (Saturday night palsy), needle examination may show neurogenic changes when compression at the spiral groove produces axonal loss.

In a posterior interosseous nerve lesion, needle examination may show neurogenic changes when pathology produces axonal loss.

Extensor Carpi Ulnaris

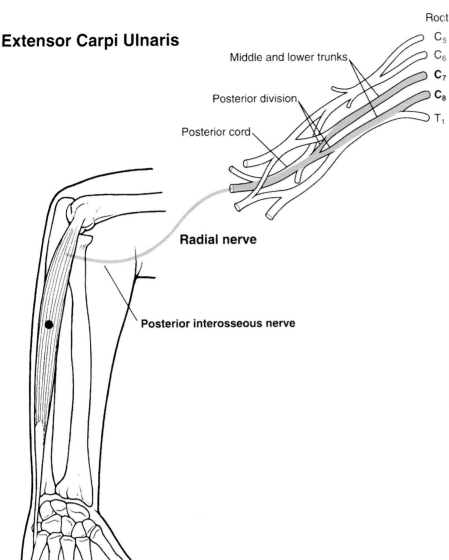

Root
C₅
C₆
C₇
C₈
T₁

Middle and lower trunks

Posterior division

Posterior cord

Radial nerve

Posterior interosseous nerve

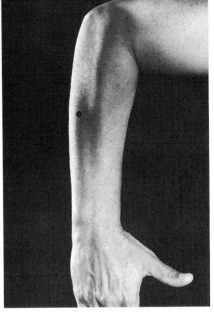

Innervation
Innervation is via the posterior interosseous nerve, radial nerve, posterior cord, middle and lower trunks, and roots C_7, C_8.

Origin
The extensor carpi ulnaris originates at the common extensor tendon from the lateral epicondyle of the humerus.

Insertion
Insertion is at the ulnar side of the base of the fifth metacarpal bone.

Activation Maneuver
Wrist extension with ulnar deviation activates the muscle.

EMG Needle Insertion
Insert the needle in the mid to upper forearm just radial to the lateral margin of the shaft of the ulna.

Pitfalls
If the needle is inserted too laterally (radially), it may be in the extensor digiti minimi or extensor digitorum communis; both are innervated by the posterior interosseous nerve.

Clinical Comments
In a radial nerve lesion at the axilla (crutch neuropathy), needle examination may show neurogenic changes when compression produces axonal loss.

In a radial nerve lesion at the upper arm (Saturday night palsy), needle examination may show neurogenic changes when compression at the spiral groove produces axonal loss.

In a posterior interosseous nerve lesion, needle examination may show neurogenic changes when pathology produces axonal loss.

Supinator

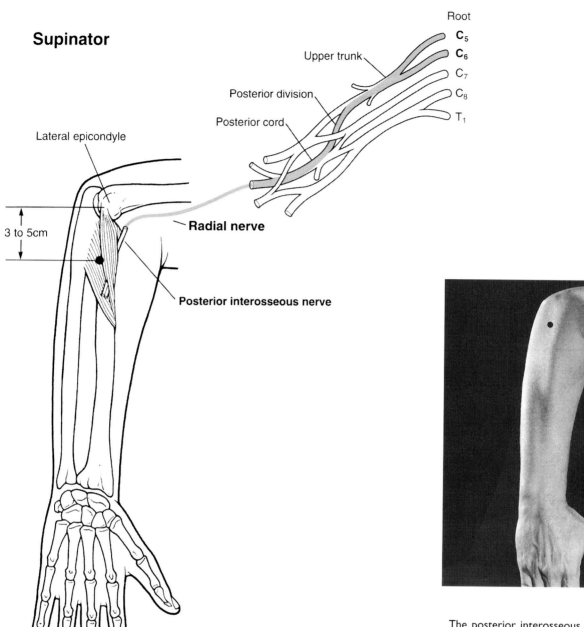

Root
C₅
C₆
C₇
C₈
T₁

Upper trunk

Posterior division

Posterior cord

Lateral epicondyle

3 to 5cm

Radial nerve

Posterior interosseous nerve

Innervation
Innervation is via the posterior interosseous nerve, radial nerve, posterior cord, upper trunk, and roots C_5, C_6.

Origin
The supinator originates at the lateral epicondyle of the humerus, radial collateral ligament of the elbow, and ridge of the ulna.

Insertion
Insertion is at the dorsal and lateral surfaces of upper third of the radius.

Activation Maneuver
Supination of the forearm activates the muscle.

EMG Needle Insertion
With the forearm pronated, insert the needle 3–5 cm distal to the lateral epicondyle, toward the shaft of the radius.

Pitfalls and Clinical Comments
This muscle lies deep. It is rarely of benefit to test it in a routine EMG evaluation.

The posterior interosseous nerve lies between the superficial and deep layers of this muscle in the arcade of Frohse. Entrapment at this site produces the posterior interosseous nerve syndrome, sometimes referred to as the *supinator syndrome*. The needle examination is usually normal. (Note: The muscle naming a syndrome is usually spared in that syndrome.)

In a radial nerve lesion at the axilla (crutch neuropathy), needle examination may show neurogenic changes when compression produces axonal loss.

In a radial nerve lesion at the upper arm (Saturday night palsy), needle examination may show neurogenic changes when compression at the spiral groove produces axonal loss.

Extensor Carpi Radialis, Longus and Brevis

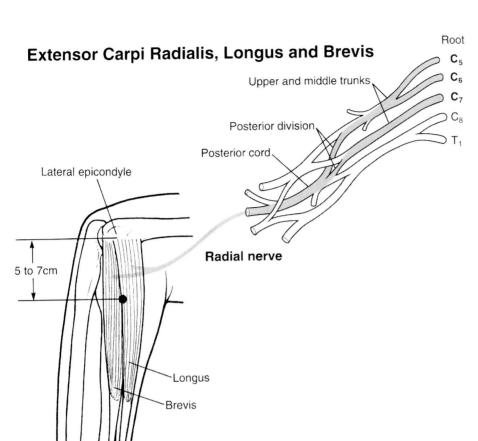

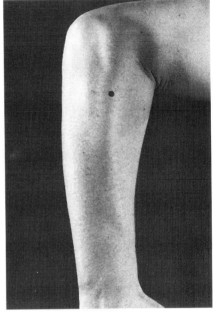

Innervation
Innervation is via the radial nerve, posterior cord, upper and middle trunks, and roots C_5, C_6, C_7.

Origin
The extensor carpi radialis longus originates at the lower third of the lateral supracondylar ridge of the humerus.

The extensor carpi radials brevis originates at the common extensor tendon from the lateral epicondyle of the humerus.

Insertion
Longus: Insertion is at the radial surface of the base of the second metacarpal bone.

Brevis: Insertion is at the radial surface of the base of the third metacarpal bone.

Activation Maneuver
Extension and radial deviation of the wrist activates the muscles. The activation maneuver should be performed while flexing the digits to avoid coactivating the extensor digitorum communis.

EMG Needle Insertion
Insert the needle in the upper forearm 5–7 cm distal to the lateral epicondyle along a line connecting the epicondyle and second metacarpal bone.

Pitfalls
If the needle is inserted too laterally (radially), it may be in the brachioradialis, which is also innervated by the radial nerve.

If the needle is inserted too medially (ulnarly), it may be in the extensor digitorum communis, which receives innervation from the posterior interosseous nerve.

Clinical Comments
In a radial nerve lesion at the axilla (crutch neuropathy), needle examination may show neurogenic changes when compression produces axonal loss.

In a radial nerve lesion at the upper arm (Saturday night palsy), needle examination may show neurogenic changes when compression at the spiral groove produces axonal loss.

In a posterior interosseous nerve lesion, needle examination will be normal.

Brachioradialis

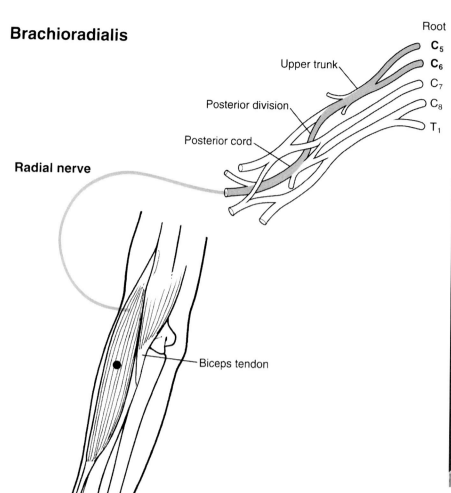

Root

C₅
C₆
C₇
C₈
T₁

Upper trunk

Posterior division

Posterior cord

Radial nerve

Biceps tendon

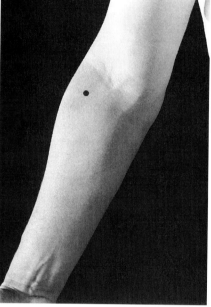

Innervation

Innervation is via the radial nerve, posterior cord, upper trunk, and roots C_5, C_6.

Origin

The brachioradialis originates at the upper two-thirds of the lateral supracondylar ridge of the humerus.

Insertion

Insertion is at the lateral aspect of the base of the styloid process of the radius.

Activation Maneuver

Flexion of the forearm in the neutral position (may act both as a supinator or pronator to bring the forearm back to a neutral position) activates the muscle.

EMG Needle Insertion

Insert the needle 2–3 cm lateral to the biceps tendon. The brachiordialis is the first muscle lateral to the biceps tendon.

Pitfalls

If the needle is inserted too laterally (radially), it may be in the extensor carpi radialis, which is also innervated by the radial nerve.

If the needle is inserted too medially (ulnarly) and distally, it may be in the pronator teres, which receives innervation from the median nerve.

Clinical Comments

This muscle is the only major flexor of the elbow joint not innervated by the musculocutaneous nerve.

In a radial nerve lesion at the axilla (crutch neuropathy), needle examination may show neurogenic changes when compression produces axonal loss.

In a radial nerve lesion at the upper arm (Saturday night palsy), needle examination may show neurogenic changes when compression at the spiral groove produces axonal loss.

In a posterior interosseous nerve lesion, needle examination will be normal.

Anconeus

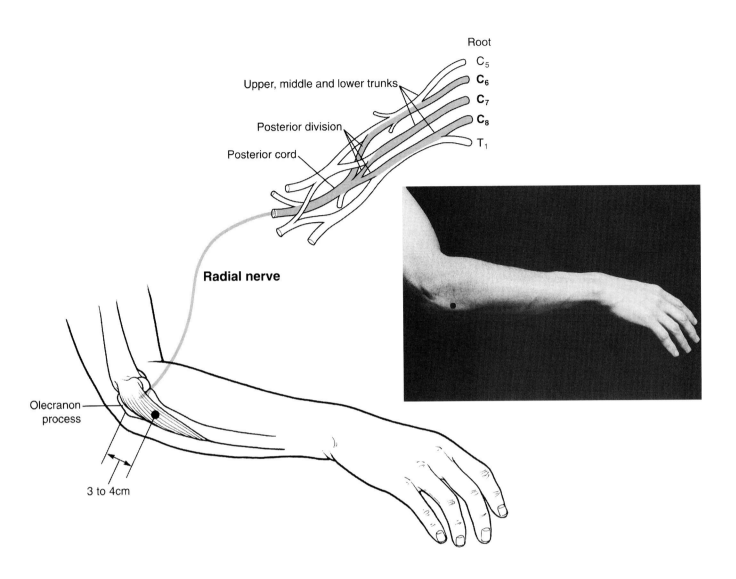

Root
C$_5$
C$_6$
C$_7$
C$_8$
T$_1$

Upper, middle and lower trunks

Posterior division

Posterior cord

Radial nerve

Olecranon
process

3 to 4cm

Innervation

Innervation is via the radial nerve; posterior cord; upper, middle, and lower trunks; and roots C$_6$, C$_7$, C$_8$

Origin

The aconeus originates at the posterior aspect of the lateral epicondyle of the humerus.

Insertion

Insertion is at the lateral aspect of the olecranon process and upper fourth of the posterior surface of the ulna.

Activation Maneuver

Extension of the forearm activates the muscle.

EMG Needle Insertion

Insert the needle 3–4 cm distal to the olecranon along the radial border of the ulna.

Pitfalls

If the needle is inserted along the medial (ulnar) border of the ulna, it may be in the flexor digitorum profundus, which is innervated by the ulnar and median nerves.

If the needle is inserted too radially or distally, it may be in the extensor carpi ulnaris, which receives innervation from the posterior interosseous nerve.

If the needle is inserted too deeply, it may be in the supinator, which receives in-

nervation from the posterior interosseous nerve.

Clinical Comments

The anconeus is a continuation of the medial head of the triceps. It is the only forearm muscle innervated by the radial nerve that is spared in lesions at the upper arm (Saturday night palsy).

In a radial nerve lesion at the axilla (crutch neuropathy), needle examination may show neurogenic changes when compression produces axonal loss.

In a posterior interosseous nerve lesion, needle examination will be normal.

Triceps, Lateral Head

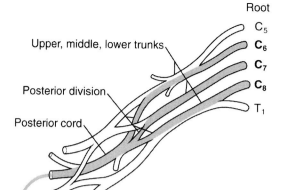

Root
C₅
C₆
C₇
C₈
T₁

Upper, middle, lower trunks

Posterior division

Posterior cord

Radial nerve

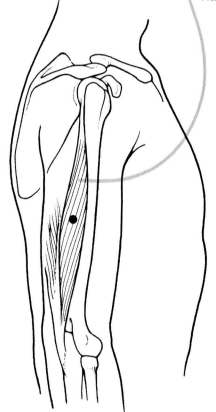

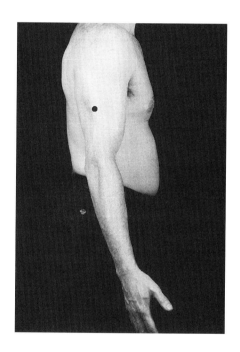

Innervation
Innervation is via the radial nerve; posterior cord; upper, middle, and lower trunks; and roots C_6, C_7, C_8.

Origin
The lateral head of the triceps originates in the posterior aspect of the shaft of the humerus.

Insertion
Insertion is at the posterior aspect of the olecranon process of the ulna.

Activation Maneuver
Extension of the forearm at the elbow joint activates the muscle.

EMG Needle Insertion
Insert the needle at the midarm level posterior to the lateral aspect of the shaft of the humerus.

Pitfalls
If the needle is inserted too proximally, it may be in the deltoid, which is innervated by the axillary nerve.

If the needle is inserted too anteriorly, it may be in the lateral border of the brachialis or biceps, which are innervated by the musculocutaneous nerve.

Clinical Comments
In a radial nerve lesion at the upper arm (Saturday night palsy), needle examination is almost always normal.

In a radial nerve lesion at the axilla (crutch neuropathy), needle examination may show neurogenic changes when compression produces axonal loss.

In a posterior interosseous nerve lesion, needle examination will be normal.

Triceps, Long Head

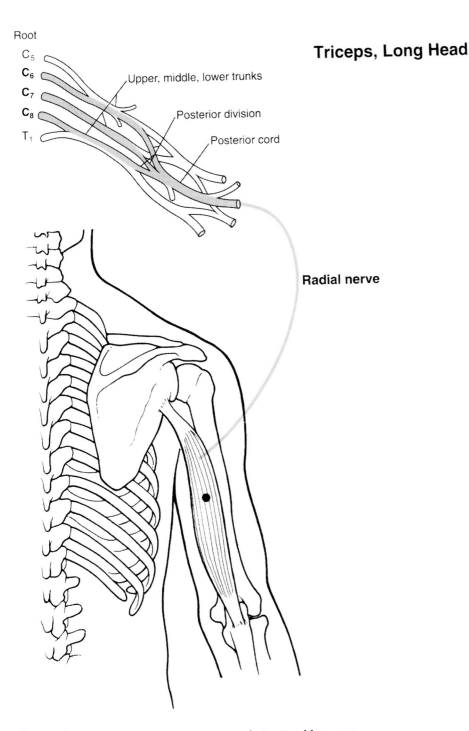

Root
C₅
C₆
C₇
C₈
T₁

Upper, middle, lower trunks

Posterior division

Posterior cord

Radial nerve

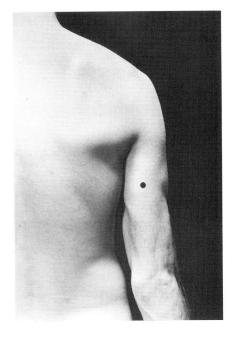

Innervation
Innervation is via the radial nerve; posterior cord; upper, middle, and lower trunks; and roots C_6, C_7, C_8.

Origin
The long head of the triceps originates at the scapula, immediately below the glenoid cavity.

Insertion
Insertion is at the posterior aspect of the olecranon process of the ulna.

Activation Maneuver
Extension of the forearm at the elbow joint activates the muscle.

EMG Needle Insertion
Insert the needle into the posterior aspect of the arm in the midline, at the junction of the upper and middle thirds of the arm.

Pitfalls
If the needle is inserted too proximally, it may be in the posterior head of the deltoid, which is innervated by the axillary nerve.

Clinical Comments
In a radial nerve lesion at the upper arm (Saturday night palsy), needle examination is almost always normal.

In a radial nerve lesion at the axilla (crutch neuropathy), needle examination may show neurogenic changes when compression produces axonal loss.

In a posterior interosseous nerve lesion, needle examination will be normal.

Triceps, Medial Head

Root
C₅
C₆
C₇
C₈
T₁

Upper, middle, lower trunks

Posterior division

Posterior cord

Radial nerve

4 to 5cm

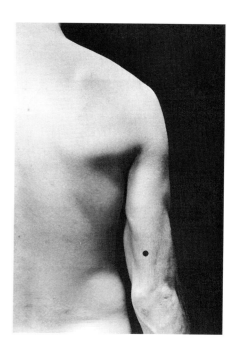

There is a risk of entering the ulnar or median nerves or of puncturing the brachial artery.

Innervation

Innervation is via the radial nerve; posterior cord; upper, middle, and lower trunks; and roots C₆, C₇, C₈.

Origin

The medial head originates in the posterior surface of the shaft of the humerus, below the spiral groove.

Insertion

Insertion is at the posterior aspect of the olecranon process of the ulna.

Activation Maneuver

Extension of the forearm at the elbow joint activates the muscle.

EMG Needle Insertion

Insert the needle 4–5 cm proximal to the olecranon process just medial to the shaft of the humerus.

Pitfalls

If the needle is inserted too anteriorly, it may be in the medial border of the brachialis or biceps, which are innervated by the musculocutaneous nerve.

Clinical Comments

Testing the medial head of the triceps is rarely of benefit in a routine EMG needle evaluation.

In a radial nerve lesion at the upper arm (Saturday night palsy), needle examination is almost always normal.

In a radial nerve lesion at the axilla (crutch neuropathy), needle examination may show neurogenic changes when compression produces axonal loss.

In a posterior interosseous nerve lesion, needle examination will be normal.

chapter
5

Axillary

Nerve

AXILLARY NERVE

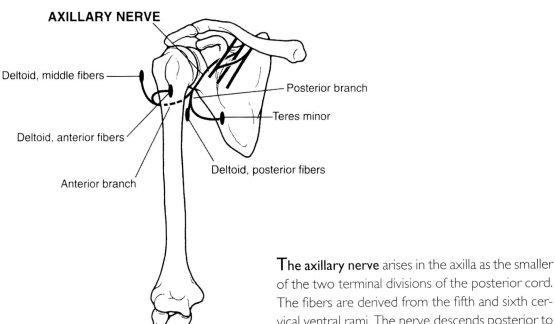

Deltoid, middle fibers ——

Deltoid, anterior fibers

Anterior branch

Posterior branch

Teres minor

Deltoid, posterior fibers

Diagram of the axillary nerve and the muscles
that it supplies.

The axillary nerve arises in the axilla as the smaller
of the two terminal divisions of the posterior cord.
The fibers are derived from the fifth and sixth cervical ventral rami. The nerve descends posterior to
the axillary artery and anterior to the subscapularis
muscle. At the lower border of the subscapularis,
it curves posteriorly through the quadrangular
space with the capsule of the shoulder joint above
(humeroscapular articular capsule), the surgical
neck of the humerus laterally, the long head of the
triceps medially, and the teres major below. In this
part of its course it is accompanied by the posterior
circumflex artery.

As the nerve emerges from the quadrangular
space, it divides into anterior and posterior terminal
divisions. The posterior branch deviates medially

and supplies the teres minor and the posterior fibers of the deltoid, which take origin from the spine of the scapula. It then gives off a branch, the upper lateral cutaneous nerve of the arm, to reach and ramify over the skin superficial to the deltoid. The anterior branch turns laterally around the surgical neck of the humerus, accompanied by the posterior circumflex artery. It then supplies the middle and anterior fibers of the deltoid, which take origin from the acromion and clavicle, respectively.

AXILLARY NERVE LESION

Etiology

An axillary nerve lesion can occur secondary to inferior dislocation of the humerus at the shoulder joint (the nerve is stretched across the head of the humerus).

An axillary nerve lesion can occur secondary to fractures of the surgical neck of the humerus.

Deep penetrating wounds and upward pressure in the axilla from misused crutches, which also compress the radial nerve (Sunderland, 1968), can cause an axillary nerve lesion.

Neuralgic amyotrophy (brachial plexopathy) can be causative.

General Comments

The most common lesions are those associated with injuries about the shoulder joint.

Clinical Features

Wasting and weakness of the deltoid are present. In the early stages following injury, the arm may hang uselessly by the side. Later, the supplementary actions of other shoulder girdle muscles, including supraspinatus, may result in abduction of the arm even in the absence of deltoid function (Sunderland, 1968).

There is a patch of sensory loss over the outer aspect of the upper arm.

Weakness of the teres minor is not easily demonstrated because other unaffected muscles, such as the infraspinatus, perform the same action.

Most lesions resolve spontaneously.

Electrodiagnostic Strategy

Demonstrate neurogenic EMG changes limited to the deltoid and teres minor.

EMG of nonaxillary innervated C_5, C_6 muscles may be necessary to exclude cervical radiculopathy.

Motor conduction studies may show reduced amplitude on the affected side.

REFERENCES

Gray's Anatomy. 38th Edition. Churchill Livingstone, New York, 1995, pp 1266–1274.

Kimura J: Electrodiagnosis in Diseases of Nerve and Muscle. 2nd Edition. FA Davis, Philadelphia, 1989, p 499.

Sunderland S: Nerves and Nerve Injuries. Williams & Wilkins, Baltimore, 1968, pp 939–945.

Deltoid, Anterior Fibers

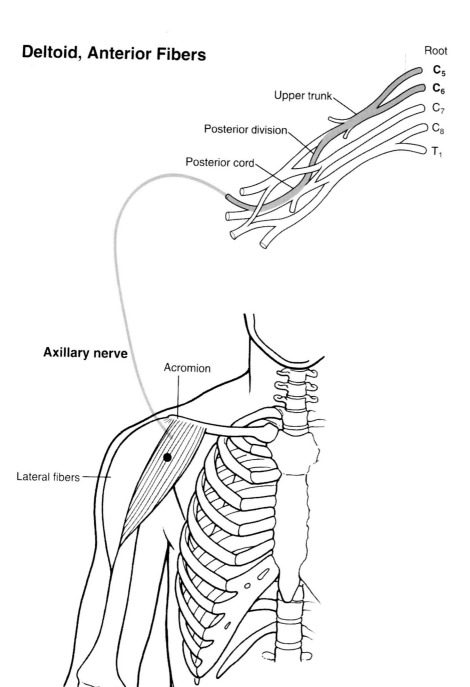

Root
C₅
C₆
C₇
C₈
T₁

Upper trunk

Posterior division

Posterior cord

Axillary nerve

Acromion

Lateral fibers

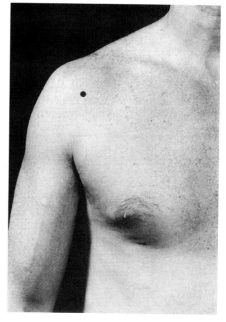

the short head of the biceps. These muscles are supplied by the musculocutaneous nerve.

If the needle is inserted too medially, it may be in the clavicular portion of the pectoralis major, supplied by the medial and lateral pectoral nerves.

Innervation

Innervation is via the axillary nerve, posterior cord, upper trunk and roots C_5, C_6.

Origin

The anterior fibers of the deltoid originate at the anterior border and superior surface of the lateral third of the clavicle.

Insertion

Insertion is at the deltoid tuberosity on the lateral aspect of the humerus midshaft.

Activation Maneuver

Forward flexion and medial rotation of the arm activate the anterior fibers of the deltoid (the anterior fibers are assisted by the pectoralis major and coracobrachialis).

EMG Needle Insertion

Insert the needle 3–4 cm directly beneath the anterior margin of the acromion.

Pitfalls

If the needle is inserted too deeply, it may be in the coracobrachialis or tendon of

Clinical Comments

Needle examination may show neurogenic changes when injury to the axillary nerve produces axonal loss (i.e., blunt trauma, fracture or dislocation of the head of the humerus, brachial plexopathy).

In C_5, C_6 radiculopathy, needle examination may show neurogenic changes when root pathology has resulted in axonal loss (i.e., in moderate to severe radiculopathy).

In Erb's palsy (C_5, C_6 root avulsion), needle examination will show neurogenic changes.

Deltoid, Middle Fibers

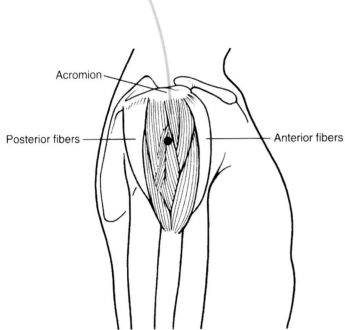

Root
- C₅
- C₆
- C₇
- C₈
- T₁

Upper trunk
Posterior division
Posterior cord

Axillary nerve

Acromion
Posterior fibers
Anterior fibers

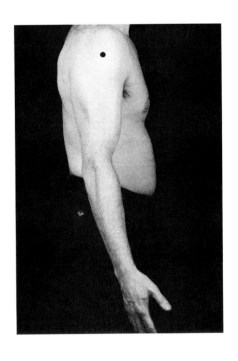

Innervation
Innervation is via the axillary nerve, posterior cord, upper trunk, and roots C₅, C₆.

Origin
The middle fibers of the deltoid originate in the lateral margin and superior surface of the acromion.

Insertion
Insertion is at the deltoid tuberosity on the lateral aspect of the humerus midshaft.

Activation Maneuver
Abduction of the arm activates the middle fibers of the deltoid (the middle fibers are assisted by the supraspintus).

EMG Needle Insertion
Insert the needle 4–5 cm directly beneath the lateral border of the acromion.

Pitfalls
There are no pitfalls.

Clinical Comments
Needle examination may show neurogenic changes when injury to the axillary nerve produces axonal loss (i.e., blunt trauma, fracture or dislocation of the head of the humerus, brachial plexopathy).

A history of multiple intramuscular injections into this muscle may confound needle findings.

In C₅, C₆ radiculopathy, needle examination may show neurogenic changes when root pathology has resulted in axonal loss (i.e., in moderate to severe radiculopathy).

In Erb's palsy (C₅, C₆ root avulsion), needle examination will show neurogenic changes.

Deltoid, Posterior Fibers

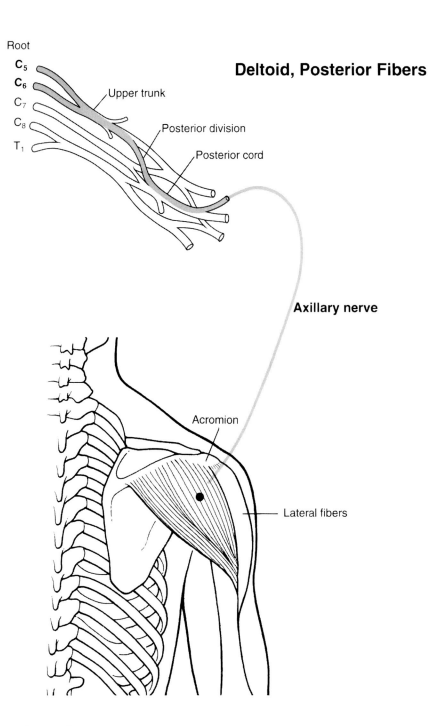

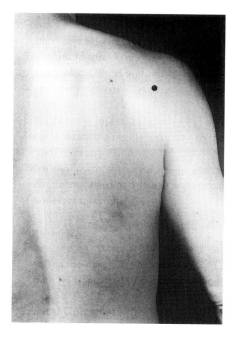

Root
C₅
C₆
C₇
C₈
T₁

Upper trunk

Posterior division

Posterior cord

Axillary nerve

Acromion

Lateral fibers

of the triceps, which are innervated by the axillary and radial nerves, respectively.

If the needle is inserted too medially, it may be in the infraspinatus, which is innervated by the suprascapular nerve.

Innervation
Innervation is via the axillary nerve, posterior cord, upper trunk, and roots C₅, C₆.

Origin
The posterior fibers of the deltoid originate at the lower edge of the crest of the spine of the scapula.

Insertion
Insertion is at the deltoid tuberosity of the humerus.

Activation Maneuver
Backward extension and lateral rotation of the arm activate the posterior fibers of the deltoid (the posterior fibers are assisted in backward extension by the latissimus dorsi and teres major).

EMG Needle Insertion
Insert the needle 3–4 cm directly beneath the posterior margin of the acromion.

Pitfalls
If the needle is inserted too deeply, it may be in the teres minor or the long head

Clinical Comments
Needle examination may show neurogenic changes when injury to the axillary nerve produces axonal loss, (i.e., blunt trauma, fracture or dislocation of the head of the humerus, brachial plexopathy).

In C₅, C₆ radiculopathy, needle examination may show neurogenic changes when root pathology has resulted in axonal loss (i.e., in moderate to severe radiculopathy).

In Erb's palsy (C₅, C₆ root avulsion), needle examination will show neurogenic changes.

Teres Minor

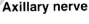

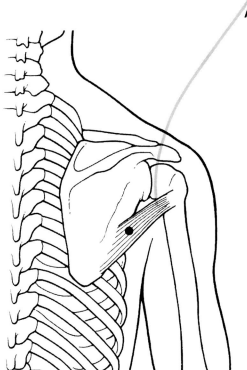

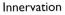

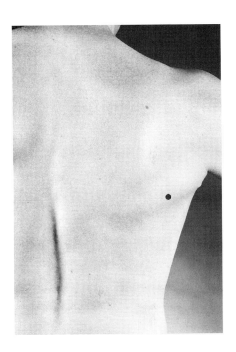

If the needle is inserted too medially or rostrally, it may be in the infraspinatus, which is innervated by the suprascapular nerve. (Note: The teres minor is sometimes fused with the infraspinatus.)

Innervation

Innervation is via the axillary nerve, posterior cord, upper trunk, and roots C_5, C_6.

Origin

The teres minor originates in the upper two-thirds of the dorsolateral surface of the scapula.

Insertion

Insertion is at the lowest facet on the greater tubercle of the humerus.

Activation Maneuver

Lateral rotation of the arm (assisted by infraspinatus and posterior fibers of deltoid) activates the muscle.

EMG Needle Insertion

Insert the needle immediately lateral to the middle third of the lateral border of the scapula.

Pitfalls

If the needle is inserted too superficially, it may be in the posterior deltoid, which is also supplied by the axillary nerve.

Clinical Comments

Needle examination may show neurogenic changes when injury to the axillary nerve produces axonal loss (i.e., blunt trauma, fracture or dislocation of the head of the humerus, brachial plexopathy).

In C_5, C_6 radiculopathy, needle examination may show neurogenic changes when root pathology has resulted in axonal loss (i.e., in moderate to severe radiculopathy).

In Erb's palsy (C_5, C_6 root avulsion), needle examination will show neurogenic changes.

chapter
6

Musculocutaneous

Nerve

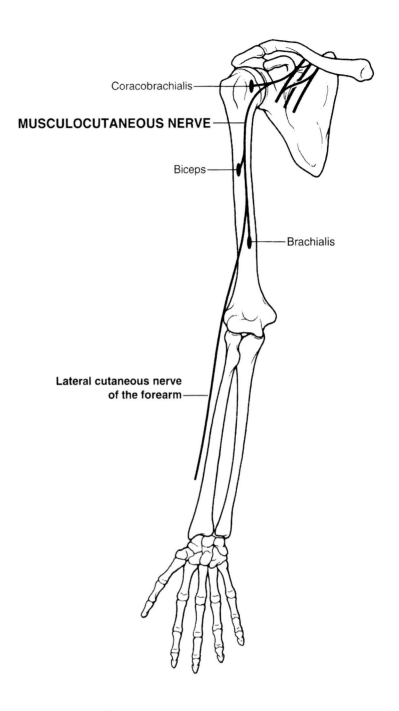

Coracobrachialis

MUSCULOCUTANEOUS NERVE

Biceps

Brachialis

**Lateral cutaneous nerve
of the forearm**

Diagram of the musculocutaneous nerve and the
muscles that it supplies.

Fibers to the musculocutaneous nerve are derived primarily from the fifth and sixth cervical roots, with an occasional contribution from the seventh cervical root (Gray's Anatomy, 1995). The nerve trunk arises from the lateral cord of the brachial plexus near the lower border of the pectoralis minor muscle. It proceeds downward to pierce the coracobrachialis muscle, which it innervates. The nerve passes through this muscle to reach the interval between the brachialis and biceps muscles. The nerve supplies both of these muscles as it descends between them. Just below the elbow it pierces the deep fascia lateral to the tendon of the biceps, continuing as the *lateral cutaneous nerve of the forearm*. This branch provides cutaneous innervation to the lateral aspect of the forearm, as far as the midline anteriorly and posteriorly, and as distal as the base of the thenar eminence and dorsolateral aspect of the wrist (Sunderland, 1968).

MUSCULOCUTANEOUS NERVE LESION

Etiology

Trauma and deep penetrating wounds can cause a musculocutaneous lesion.

Neuralgic amyotrophy (idiopathic brachial plexopathy) can be causative.

Rarely, entrapment of the musculocutaneous nerve as it passes through the coracobrachialis (Braddom and Wolfe, 1978) can cause a musculocutaneous lesion.

General Comments

Trauma almost always results in combined lesions of the musculocutaneous nerve and the lateral cord of the brachial plexus (Sunderland, 1968).

Clinical Features

Wasting and weakness of the coracobrachialis, biceps, and brachialis can occur. In complete lesions of the musculocutaneous nerve, the supinator and brachioradialis hypertrophy and may compensate for the loss of the biceps and brachialis muscles.

Loss of the biceps tendon reflex occurs.

There is sensory loss over the lateral aspect of the forearm.

Electrodiagnostic Strategy

Demonstrate neurogenic EMG changes in the coracobrachialis, biceps, and brachialis.

EMG of other C_5 and C_6 muscles may be necessary to exclude cervical radiculopathy.

Musculocutaneous motor conduction studies may show reduced amplitude or absence on the affected side.

Sensory conduction studies of the lateral cutaneous nerve of the forearm may show reduced amplitude or absence on the affected side.

REFERENCES

Braddom R L, Wolfe C: Musculocutaneous nerve injury after heavy exercise. Arch Phys Med Rehabil 1978;59:290–293.

Gray's Anatomy. 38th Edition. Churchill Livingstone, New York, 1995, pp 1266–1274.

Sunderland S: Nerves and Nerve Injuries. Williams & Wilkins, Baltimore, 1968, pp 886–893.

Brachialis

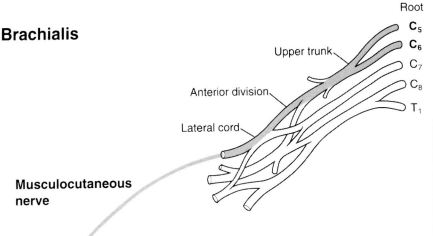

Root
C₅
C₆
C₇
C₈
T₁

Upper trunk

Anterior division

Lateral cord

Musculocutaneous nerve

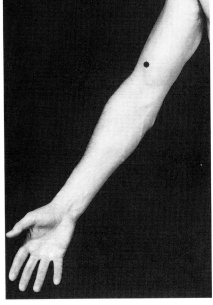

Innervation

Innervation is via the musculocutaneous nerve, lateral cord, upper trunk, and roots C_5, C_6. Note: A small lateral portion of the muscle may receive radial nerve innervation (C_7 root).

Origin

The brachialis originates in the lower half of the anterior surface of the humerus.

Insertion

Insertion is at the ulnar tuberosity and the anterior part of the coronoid process of the ulna.

Activation Maneuver

Flexion of the forearm at the elbow activates the muscle.

EMG Needle Insertion

Lateral approach: Insert the needle 4–5 cm proximal to the elbow crease just lateral to and under the biceps.

Medial approach: This approach is not recommended because it risks injury to the median nerve, brachial artery, and basilic vein.

Pitfalls

If the needle is inserted too distally and posteriorly, it may be in the proximal brachioradialis or extensor carpi radialis longus; these muscles are supplied by the radial nerve.

If the needle is inserted too proximal and posteriorly, it may be in the lateral head of the triceps, which is supplied by the radial nerve.

Clinical Comments

Needle examination may show neurogenic changes when injury to the musculocutaneous nerve produces axonal loss.

In brachial plexopathy, needle examination may show neurogenic changes when lateral cord pathology has resulted in axonal loss.

In C_5, C_6 radiculopathy, needle examination may show neurogenic changes when root pathology has resulted in axonal loss (i.e., in moderate to severe radiculopathy).

In Erb's palsy (C_5, C_6 root avulsion), needle examination will show neurogenic changes.

Biceps Brachii

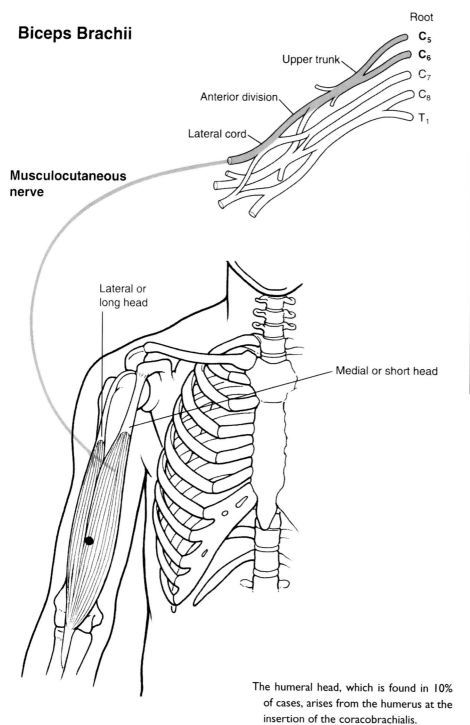

Root
C₅
C₆
C₇
C₈
T₁

Upper trunk

Anterior division

Lateral cord

Musculocutaneous nerve

Lateral or long head

Medial or short head

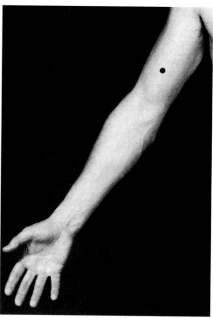

EMG Needle Insertion
Insert the needle into the midarm anteriorly, into bulk of the muscle.

Pitfalls
If the needle is inserted too proximally, it may be in the anterior deltoid (supplied by the axillary nerve) or the pectoralis major (supplied by the medial and lateral pectoral nerves).

If the needle is inserted too deeply, it may be in the brachialis, which is also supplied by the musculocutaneous nerve.

Clinical comments
Needle examination may show neurogenic changes when injury to the musculocutaneous nerve produces axonal loss.

In brachial plexopathy, needle examination may show neurogenic changes when lateral cord pathology has resulted in axonal loss.

In C_5, C_6 radiculopathy, needle examination may show neurogenic changes when root pathology has resulted in axonal loss (i.e., in moderate to severe radiculopathy).

In Erb's palsy (C_5, C_6 root avulsion), needle examination will show neurogenic changes.

The humeral head, which is found in 10% of cases, arises from the humerus at the insertion of the coracobrachialis.

Innervation
Innervation is via the musculocutaneous nerve, lateral cord, upper trunk, and roots C_5, C_6.

Origin
The medial or short head of the biceps brachii originates at the coracoid process of the scapula.

The lateral or long head originates at the supraglenoid tubercle of the scapula.

Insertion
Insertion is at the posterior aspect of the radial tuberosity (the tuberosity lies distal to the medial part of the neck of the radius).

Activation Maneuver
Flexion and supination of the forearm at the elbow activates the biceps brachii. To a slight extent, the biceps also acts to flex the arm at the shoulder.

Coracobrachialis

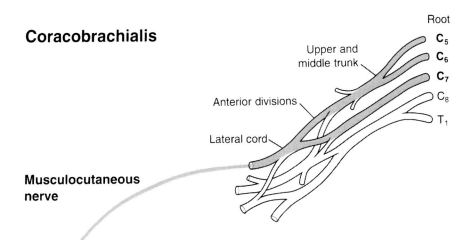

Root
C₅
C₆
C₇
C₈
T₁

Upper and middle trunk

Anterior divisions

Lateral cord

Musculocutaneous nerve

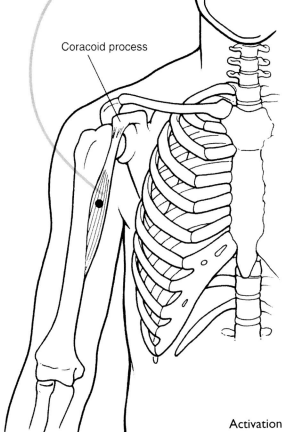

Coracoid process

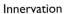

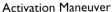

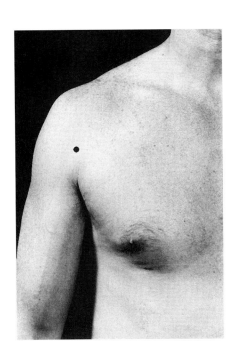

Innervation
Innervation is via the musculocutaneous nerve, lateral cord, upper and middle trunks, and roots C_5, C_6, C_7.

Origin
The coracobrachialis originates at the apex of the coracoid process of the scapula.

Insertion
Insertion is at the medial surface of the shaft of the humerus.

Activation Maneuver
Forward elevation of the humerus activates the muscle. The coracobrachialis stabilizes the head of the humerus in relation to the glenoid fossa of the scapula.

EMG Needle Insertion
Insert the needle 6–8 cm distal to the coracoid process along the volar aspect of the arm.

Pitfalls
If the needle is inserted too laterally and superficially, it may be in the short head of the biceps, which is also innervated by the musculocutaneous nerve.

If the needle is inserted too proximal and superficial, it may be in the anterior deltoid, which is supplied by the axillary nerve.

Clinical Comments
Needle examination may show neurogenic changes when injury to the musculocutaneous nerve produces axonal loss.

In brachial plexopathy, needle examination may show neurogenic changes when lateral cord pathology has resulted in axonal loss.

In C_5, C_6, C_7 radiculopathy, needle examination may show neurogenic changes when root pathology has resulted in axonal loss (i.e., in moderate to severe radiculopathy).

chapter
7

Suprascapular

Nerve

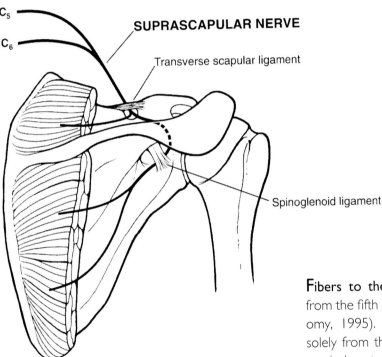

C₅
C₆

SUPRASCAPULAR NERVE

Transverse scapular ligament

Spinoglenoid ligament

Diagram of the suprascapular nerve (posterior view) to the supraspinatus and infraspinatus muscles.

Fibers to the suprascapular nerve are derived from the fifth and sixth cervical roots (Gray's Anatomy, 1995). Occasionally, the nerve is derived solely from the fifth or from the fifth and fourth cervical roots (Sunderland, 1968). The nerve arises from the upper trunk of the brachial plexus and passes obliquely outward beneath the trapezius and omohyoid muscles to reach the suprascapular notch of the scapula. This notch is bridged by the superior transverse scapular ligament to form an osseofibrous foramen through which the suprascapular nerve passes to enter the supraspinous fossa. In the fossa, the nerve lies beneath the supraspinatus muscle, which it innervates.

The nerve then continues around the curved free lateral border of the spine of the scapula to reach the spinoglenoid notch. This notch is covered by the inferior transverse scapular (or spinoglenoid) ligament, which may also form an osseofibrous foramen through which the suprascapular nerve passes to enter the infraspinous fossa. In this fossa, the nerve supplies the infraspinatus muscle. One of the most important uses of the supraspinatus- and infraspinatus muscles is the protection they afford to the shoulder joint; the supraspinatus supports it above and prevents displacement of the head of the humerus upward, while the infraspinatus (and teres minor) protect it posteriorly and prevent dislocation backward.

SUPRASCAPULAR NERVE LESION

Etiology

Trauma to the shoulder, fractures of the scapula or humerus, and penetrating wounds can cause direct nerve injury (Hadley et al., 1986).

Entrapment at the suprascapular notch of the scapula, or rarely at the spinoglenoid notch (Aiello et al., 1982), can cause a suprascapular nerve lesion.

Neuralgic amyotrophy (brachial plexopathy) is causative.

General Comments

Trauma often results in combined lesions of the suprascapular nerve and the upper trunk of the brachial plexus (Sunderland, 1968).

Clinical Features

The shoulder pain is usually described as a deep, dull ache located posterolaterally in the shoulder.

There is wasting of the supraspinatus and infraspinatus muscles.

Initiation of abduction of the arm may be difficult, and there may be weakness during external rotation of the humerus. The deltoid and teres minor usually compensate for the loss of the supraspinatus and infraspinatus muscles, respectively.

There is no sensory loss.

Electrodiagnostic Strategy

Demonstrate neurogenic EMG changes in the supraspinatus and infraspinatus muscles.

EMG of the nonsuprascapular innervated C_5, C_6 muscles may be necessary to exclude radiculopathy or coexisting upper trunk lesion.

Perform nerve conduction studies to exclude neuralgic amyotrophy.

REFERENCES

Aiello I, Serra G, Traina G C, Tugnoli V: Entrapment of the suprascapular nerve at the spinoglenoid notch. Ann Neurol 1982; 12:314–316

Gray's Anatomy. 38th Edition. Churchill Livingstone, New York, 1995, pp 1266–1274.

Hadley M N, Sonntag V K H, Pittman H W: Suprascapular nerve entrapment. J Neurosurg 1986;64:843–848.

Reinstein L, Twardzik F G, Mech K F: Pneumothorax: A complication of needle electromyography of the supraspinatus muscle. Arch Phys Med Rehabil: 1987;68: 561–562.

Sunderland S: Nerves and Nerve Injuries. Williams & Wilkins, Baltimore, 1968, pp 1119–1120.

Infraspinatus

C_5
C_6
C_7
C_8
T_1

Upper trunk

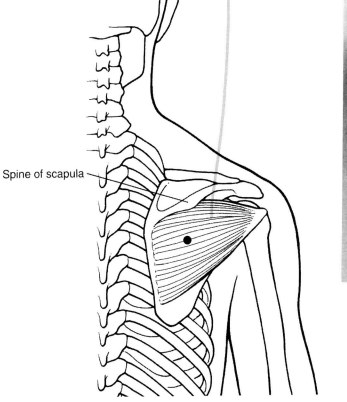

Suprascapular nerve

Spine of scapula

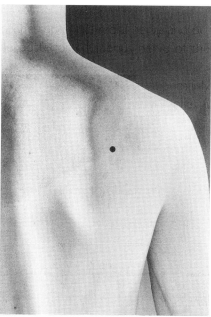

Innervation

Innervation is via the suprascapular nerve, upper trunk, and roots C_5, C_6.

Origin

The infraspinatus originates in the infraspinous fossa of the scapula.

Insertion

Insertion is at the greater tuberosity of the humerus.

Activation Maneuver

External rotation of the humerus activates the muscle.

EMG Needle Insertion

Insert the needle into the infraspinous fossa 2–4 cm below the medial one-third of the spine of the scapula.

Pitfalls

If the needle is inserted too laterally or superficially, it may be in the posterior deltoid, which is supplied by the axillary nerve. Additionally, the trapezius (which is supplied by the spinal accessory nerve) and the latissimus dorsi (supplied by the thoracodorsal nerve) may each lie superficial to the upper and lower margins of the infraspinatus muscle, respectively.

If the needle is placed too caudad, it may be in the teres minor (which is supplied by the axillary nerve) or, rarely, the teres major (supplied by the subscapular nerve).

Clinical Comments

Needle examination may show neurogenic changes when injury to the suprascapular nerve produces axonal loss.

Needle examination may also show neurogenic changes in lesions of the upper trunk and the C_5, C_6 including Erb's palsy.

Supraspinatus

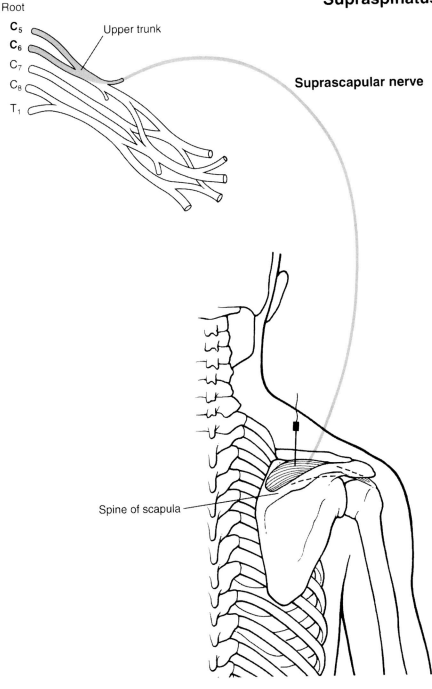

Root

C₅
C₆
C₇
C₈
T₁

Upper trunk

Suprascapular nerve

Spine of scapula

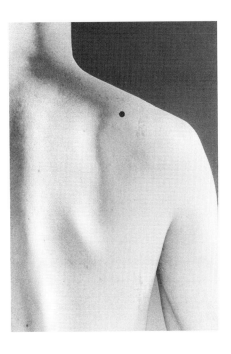

Innervation
Innervation is via the Suprascapular nerve, upper trunk, and roots C_5, C_6.

Origin
The supraspinatus originates in the supraspinous fossa of the scapula.

Insertion
Insertion is at the greater tuberosity of the humerus.

Activation Maneuver
Initiation of abduction of the arm activates the muscle.

EMG Needle Insertion
Insert the needle into the supraspinous fossa just above the spine of the scapula (the lateral margin of the spine is usually easier to palpate). Direct the needle to the bone and then retract slightly.

Pitfalls
If the needle is inserted too superficially, it will be in the trapezius muscle, which is supplied by the spinal accessory nerve and C_3 and C_4 spinal nerves.

Pneumothorax following supraspinatus EMG needle examination has been reported in the literature (Reinstein et al., 1987).

Clinical Comments
Needle examination may show neurogenic changes when injury to the suprascapular nerve produces axonal loss.

Needle examination may also show neurogenic changes in lesions of the upper trunk and C_5, C_6 roots, including Erb's palsy.

chapter

8

Dorsal Scapular

Nerve

The dorsal scapular nerve originates predominantly from the fifth cervical spinal nerve within the substance of the scalenus medius muscle, but it may receive additional fibers from the fourth and sixth spinal nerves. (Gray's Anatomy, 1995). It may arise in conjunction with the upper root of the long thoracic nerve (Sunderland, 1968). The nerve courses behind the brachial plexus and descends obliquely through the scalenus medius to reach the deep surface of the levator scapulae muscle. It usually sends a twig to this muscle, which receives most of its nerve supply from the third and fourth cervical roots. The nerve continues downward along the medial margin of the scapula to innervate the rhomboideus major and rhomboideus minor muscles (rhomboids).

DORSAL SCAPULAR NERVE LESION

Etiology

Trauma to the back and penetrating wounds can cause direct nerve injury.

Rarely, entrapment due to hypertrophy of the scalenus medius muscle (Kopell and Thompson, 1976) causes a dorsal scapular nerve lesion.

General Comments

Isolated lesions of this nerve are rare.

Clinical Features

Possible shoulder pain is most marked along the medial border of the scapula.

Wasting of the rhomboid muscles produces slight winging of the scapula.

There is difficulty drawing the scapula directly backward toward the spine. It is questionable whether an isolated nerve lesion would be clinically recognized (Sunderland, 1968) because the trapezius muscle will compensate for paralysis of the rhomboids and levator scapulae.

Electrodiagnostic Strategy

Demonstrate neurogenic EMG changes in the rhomboids and levator scapulae.

Exclude C_5 radiculopathy by performing EMG in other C_5 muscles. Note: Because isolated lesions of this nerve are rare, neurogenic EMG changes in rhomboids or levator scapulae usually imply C_5 radiculopathy.

Perform nerve conduction studies to exclude an upper trunk lesion.

REFERENCES

Gray's Anatomy. 38th Edition. Churchill Livingstone, New York, 1995, pp 835–838.

Kopell HP, Thompson WAL: Peripheral Entrapment Neuropathies. 2nd Edition. Robert E. Krieger Publishing, New York, 1976, pp 161–170.

Miller J: Pneumothorax complication of needle EMG of thoracic wall. NJ Med 1990;87(8): 653.

Sunderland S: Nerves and Nerve Injuries. Williams & Wilkins, Baltimore, 1968, p 1120.

Rhomboideus Major and Minor

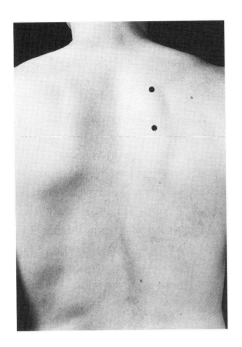

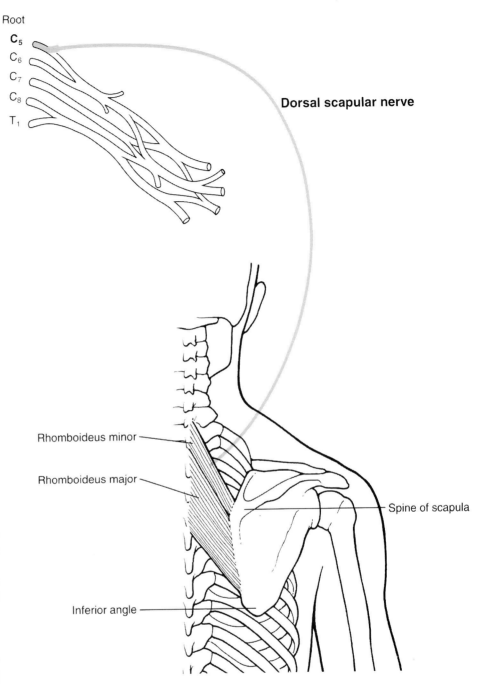

Dorsal scapular nerve

Rhomboideus minor

Rhomboideus major

Inferior angle

Spine of scapula

Innervation
Innervation is via the dorsal scapular nerve and root C_5.

Origin
The major rhomboideus originates at the spinous processes of the second to fifth thoracic vertebrae.

The minor rhomboideus originates at the spinous processes of the seventh cervical and first thoracic vertebrae.

Insertion
Major: Insertion is at the medial scapular border between the inferior angle and the spine of the scapula.

Minor: Insertion is at the medial scapular border at the base of the spine of the scapula.

Activation Maneuver
Retraction of the scapula (drawing the scapula directly backward toward the vertebral spine) activates the muscles.

EMG Needle Insertion
Major: Insert the needle just medial to the medial margin of the scapula, midway between the scapular spine and the inferior angle.

Minor: Insert the needle just medial to medial border of the scapular spine.

Pitfalls
Major and minor: If the needle is inserted too superficially, it will be in the trapezius muscle, which is supplied by the spinal accessory nerve.

Major only: If the needle is inserted too caudad and superficially, it may be in the latissimus dorsi, which is supplied by the thoracodorsal nerve.

Pneumothorax following needle examination has been reported in the literature (Miller, 1990).

Clinical Comments
Neurogenic changes in the rhomboids on needle examination usually indicate a C_5 radiculopathy.

Look for neurogenic changes in other C_5-innervated muscles.

Levator Scapulae

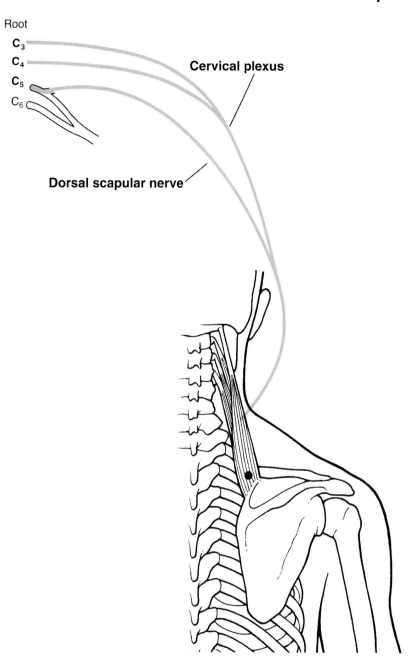

Root
C₃
C₄
C₅
C₆

Cervical plexus

Dorsal scapular nerve

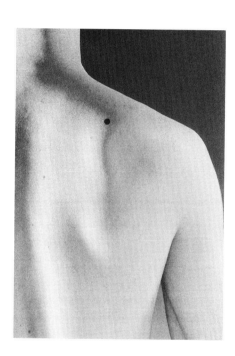

Innervation
Innervation is via the anterior rami of C₃, C₄, and C₅, the latter branch via the dorsal scapular nerve.

Origin
The levator scapulae originate at the transverse processes of the upper four cervical vertebrae.

Insertion
Insertion is at the posteromedial border of the scapula, between the superior angle and the spine of the scapula.

Activation Maneuver
Elevation of the scapula (which assists the trapezius in shrugging shoulders) activates the levator scapulae.

EMG Needle Insertion
Insert the needle along the superomedial margin of the scapula.

Pitfalls
If the needle is inserted too superficially, it will be in the trapezius muscle, which is supplied by C₃ and C₄ spinal nerves and the spinal accessory nerve.

If the needle is inserted too deeply, it may be in the paraspinal muscles, which are supplied by the posterior rami of the spinal nerves.

Clinical Comments
Neurogenic changes in this muscle on needle examination usually indicate a C₃–C₅ radiculopathy.

Look for neurogenic changes in other C₃–C₅ innervated muscles to confirm radiculopathy.

Long Thoracic

Nerve

The long thoracic nerve is formed by roots from the fifth to the seventh cervical rami (Gray's Anatomy, 1995). The upper two roots pierce the scalenus medius obliquely, unite within the muscle, and are then joined by the seventh root, which runs anterior to this muscle. The nerve descends posterior to the brachial plexus, crosses the outer border of the first rib, and descends further along the outer thoracic wall on the surface of the serratus anterior muscle. It supplies this muscle by filaments passing to the several digitations of the muscle.

LONG THORACIC NERVE LESION

Etiology
Trauma to the posterior triangle of the neck causes direct nerve injury.
Traction injury occurs when the angle between the neck and the shoulder is forcibly increased (Sunderland, 1968).

Rarely, entrapment due to hypertrophy of the scalenus medius muscle causes a long thoracic nerve lesion (Kopell and Thompson, 1976).

Neuralgic amyotrophy is causative. Winging of the scapula may be the only manifestation of neuralgic amyotrophy (Gray's Anatomy, 1995).

General Comments

Because the nerve is attached to the scalenus medius above and the serratus anterior below, the nerve is susceptible to stretch injury when the shoulder or chest wall is depressed or the neck is flexed to the opposite side.

Clinical Features

Pain that is dull aching in quality is most marked along the shoulder.

Weakness of the serratus anterior produces prominent winging of the scapula. This is easily demonstrated by asking the patient to push against resistance with the arm extended at the elbow and forward flexed to 90 degrees at the shoulder.

Electrodiagnostic Strategy

Demonstrate neurogenic EMG changes in the serratus anterior.

Exclude C_5, C_6 or C_7 radiculopathy by performing EMG in other muscles.

Perform nerve conduction studies to exclude a brachial plexus lesion.

REFERENCES

Gray's Anatomy. 38th Edition. Churchill Livingstone, New York, 1995, pp 835–838.

Johnson EW, Parker WD: Electromyography examination. In Johnson EW (ed): Practical Electromyography. Williams & Wilkins, Baltimore, 1980, pp 1–16.

Kopell HP, Thompson WAL: Peripheral Entrapment Neuropathies. 2nd Edition. Robert E. Krieger Publishing, New York, 1976, pp 167–168.

Sunderland S: Nerves and Nerve Injuries. Williams & Wilkins, Baltimore, 1968, p 1114–1117.

Serratus Anterior

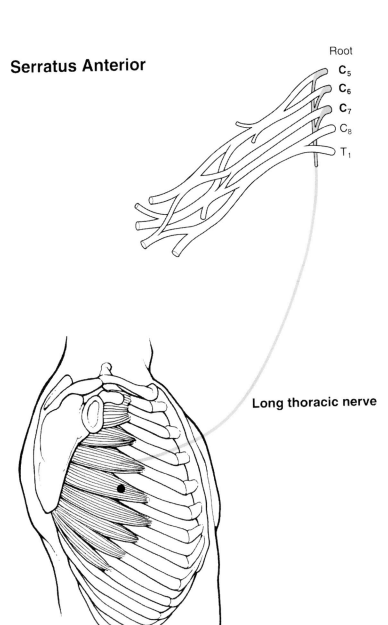

Root
C₅
C₆
C₇
C₈
T₁

Long thoracic nerve

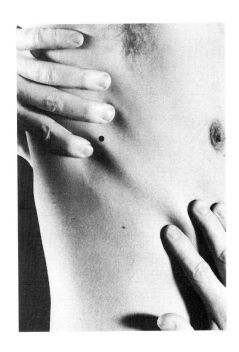

Innervation
Innervation is via the long thoracic nerve and roots C_5, C_6, C_7.

Origin
The serratus anterior originates at the outer surfaces and superior borders of the upper eight or nine ribs.

Insertion
Insertion is at the medial border of the scapula, from the superior angle to the costal surface of the inferior angle.

Activation Maneuver
Forward flexion of the arm and pushing against resistance activate the muscle.

EMG Needle Insertion
Insert the needle along the midaxillary line directly over the rib, anterior to the bulk of the latissimus dorsi but, in a woman, posterior to breast tissue. Palpating the interspace on either side can isolate a single rib. The serratus anterior is the only muscle between the skin and the rib.

Pitfalls
Pneumothorax following needle examination of the serratus anterior has been reported (Johnson and Parker, 1980).

Clinical Comments
Neurogenic EMG changes limited to the serratus anterior suggest an isolated lesion of the long thoracic nerve.
EMG of other C_5, C_6, or C_7 muscles should be performed to exclude radiculopathy.

chapter 10

Subscapular Nerves
and the
Thoracodorsal Nerve

The **subscapular nerves and the thoracodorsal nerve** are all branches of the posterior cord of the brachial plexus. The upper and lower subscapular nerves arise from the fifth and sixth cervical nerves, while the thoracodorsal nerve arises from the sixth through eighth cervical nerves. The upper and lower subscapular nerves are short and supply the subscapularis and teres major muscles, respectively (Sunderland, 1968).

The subscapularis muscle is of little EMG importance, as it is generally inaccessible to needle examination (it fills the subscapular fossa and terminates in a tendon that inserts on the lesser tuberosity of the humerus). The teres major and latissimus dorsi, however, can be examined during routine EMG evaluation. The nerve to the latissimus dorsi is historically considered as the middle or long subscapular nerve (Sunderland, 1968; Gray's Anatomy, 1977), more recently renamed the *thoracodorsal nerve* (Gray's Anatomy, 1995). The thoracodorsal nerve runs a long, exposed course on the posterior wall of the axilla to reach the deep surface of the latissimus dorsi. It is intimately related to lymph nodes along its course and may be damaged during surgical procedures on the axilla.

REFERENCES

Gray's Anatomy. 15th English Edition. Bounty Books/Crown Publishers, New York, 1977, pp 339–340.

Gray's Anatomy. 38th Edition. Churchill Livingstone, New York, 1995, pp 835–842.

Sunderland S: Nerves and Nerve Injuries. Williams & Wilkins, Baltimore, 1968, p 1120.

Teres Major

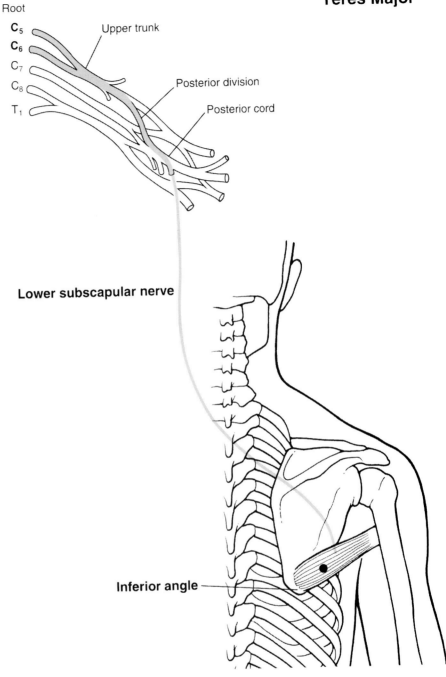

Root

C₅
C₆
C₇
C₈
T₁

Upper trunk

Posterior division

Posterior cord

Lower subscapular nerve

Inferior angle

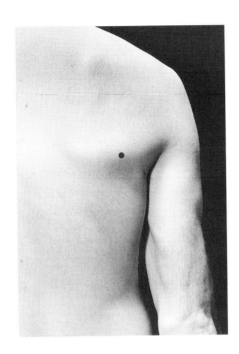

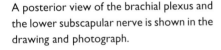

A posterior view of the brachial plexus and the lower subscapular nerve is shown in the drawing and photograph.

Innervation

Innervation is via the lower subscapular nerve, posterior cord, upper trunk, and roots C₅, C₆.

Origin

The teres major originates at the dorsal aspect of the inferior angle of the scapula.

Insertion

Insertion is at the inner bicipital ridge of the humerus.

Activation Maneuver

Internal rotation and abduction of the humerus activates the muscle.

EMG Needle Insertion

Insert the needle along the lateral lower border of the scapula (lateral and rostral to the inferior angle).

Pitfalls

If the needle is inserted too caudally or laterally, it may be in the latissimus dorsi. The latissimus at first covers the origin of the teres major and then wraps itself obliquely around its lower border so that its tendon ultimately comes to lie in front of that of the teres major.

If the needle is inserted too rostrally (superiorly), it may be in the teres minor, which is supplied by the axillary nerve.

If the needle is inserted too deeply, it may penetrate the serratus anterior, supplied by the long thoracic nerve.

Clinical Comments

An isolated lesion of the lower subscapular nerve is rare. It is unlikely that weakness limited to the teres major would be clinically detectable.

Neurogenic EMG changes in the teres major may be seen with C₅ or C₆ radiculopathy.

Latissimus Dorsi

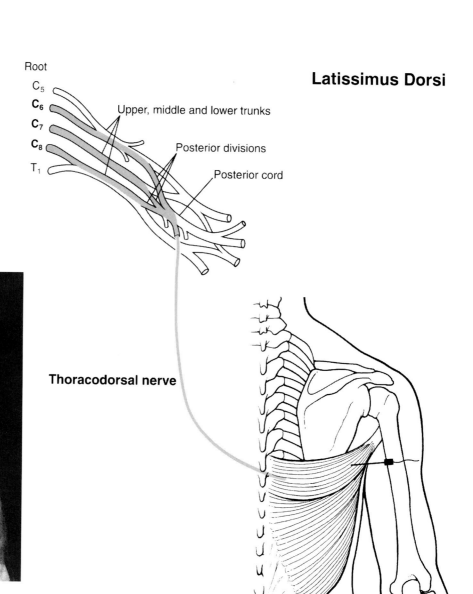

Thoracodorsal nerve

A posterior view of the brachial plexus and the thoracodorsal nerve is shown in the drawing and photograph.

Innervation
Innervation is via the thoracodorsal nerve (formerly the *middle subscapular nerve*); posterior cord; upper, middle, and lower trunks; and roots C_6, C_7, C_8.

Origin
The latissimus dorsi originates at the spinous process of the six inferior thoracic vertebrae, the posterior layer of the lumbar fascia (by which it is attached to the spines of the lumbar and sacral vertebrae), and the crest of the ilium.

Insertion
Insertion is at the bicipital groove of the humerus.

Activation Maneuver
Internal rotation, abduction, and extension (drawing the arm backward) of the humerus activates the muscle.

EMG Needle Insertion
Insert the needle along the posterior axillary fold directly lateral to the inferior angle of the scapula.

Pitfalls
If the needle is inserted too superiorly, it may be in the teres major. The latissimus at first covers the origin of the teres major and then wraps itself obliquely around its lower border so that its tendon ultimately comes to lie in front of that of the teres major.

Clinical Comments
Atrophy and weakness of the latissimus dorsi is not easily detected because wasting is not often noticeable and functions (internal rotation, adduction, and extension) can be executed by other muscles (Sunderland, 1968).

Neurogenic EMG changes in the latissimus dorsi may be seen with C_6, C_7, or C_8 radiculopathy.

chapter

11

Medial and Lateral

Pectoral Nerves

The lateral pectoral nerve is larger than the medial and arises from the upper and middle trunks or by a single branch from the lateral cord of the brachial plexus. Its fibers are derived from the fifth to seventh cervical rami (Gray's Anatomy, 1995). It crosses anterior to the axillary artery and vein, pierces the clavipectoral fascia, and supplies the deep surface of the pectoralis major. It sends a small branch to the medial pectoral nerve, forming a loop in front of the first part of the axillary artery, to supply fibers of the pectoralis minor. The medial pectoral nerve is derived from the eighth cervical and first thoracic cervical rami. It arises from the medial cord of the brachial plexus, posterior to the axillary artery. It curves forward to join the branch from the lateral pectoral nerve, entering the deep surface of the pectoralis minor to supply it. Branches from the medial pectoral nerve may also supply portions of the pectoralis major.

REFERENCES

Gray's Anatomy. 38th Edition. Churchill Livingstone, New York, 1995, pp 838–840, 1269.

Pecina M M, Krmpotic-Nemanic J, Markiewitz A D: Tunnel Syndromes: Peripheral Nerve Compression Syndromes. 2nd Edition. CRC Press, New York, 1997, pp 36–38.

Pectoralis Major

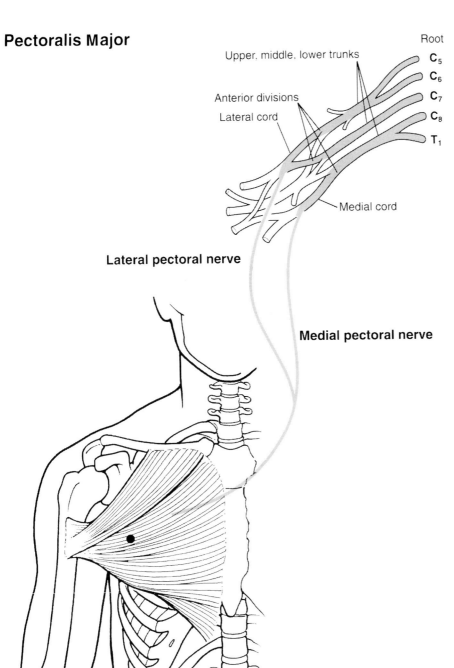

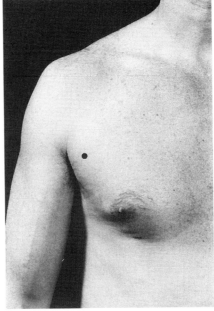

Innervation

Clavicular part: Innervation is via the lateral pectoral nerve, lateral cord, upper trunk, and roots C_5, C_6.

Sternocostal part: Innervation is via the lateral and medial pectoral nerves, lateral and medial cords, middle and lower trunks, and roots C_7, C_8, T_1.

Origin

The clavicular part originates at the sternal half of the clavicle.

The sternocostal part originates at the anterior surface of the sternum, the cartilage of the first six or seven ribs, and the aponeurosis of the external oblique muscle of the abdomen.

Insertion

Insertion is at the lateral lip of the intertubercular sulcus on the shaft of the humerus.

Activation Maneuver

Adduction of the arm activates the muscle.

EMG Needle Insertion

Insert the needle just medial to the anterior axillary fold over the bulk of the muscle.

Pitfalls

If the needle is inserted too superiorly, it may be in the anterior fibers of the deltoid, which is supplied by the axillary nerve.

If the needle is inserted too laterally, it may be in the coracobrachialis or the short head of the biceps, which are supplied by the musculocutaneous nerve.

Clinical Comments

An isolated lesion of the lateral or medial pectoral nerves is rare.

Weakness of the pectoralis major results in limited adduction of the arm.

Neurogenic EMG changes in the pectoralis major may be seen with radiculopathies affecting the C_5–T_1 roots. This muscle is therefore of little benefit in localizing a root lesion.

Pectoralis Minor

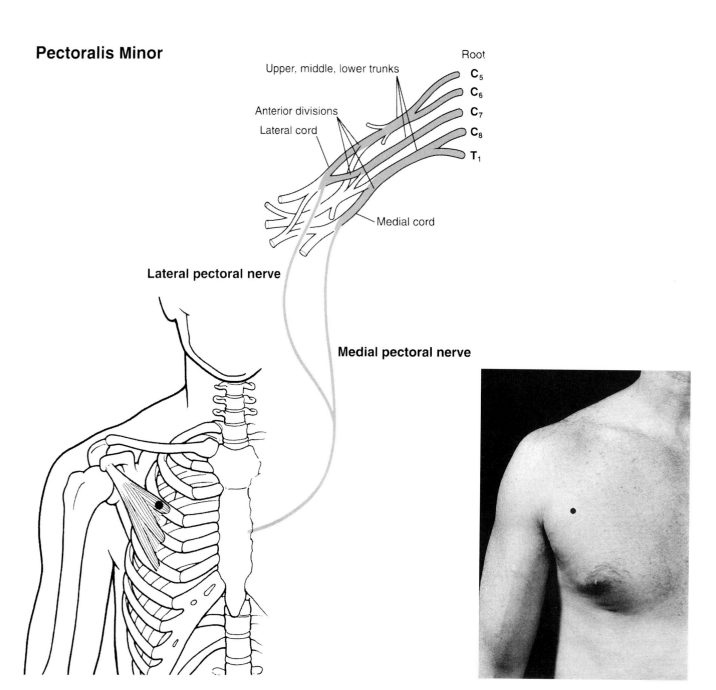

Root
C₅
C₆
C₇
C₈
T₁

Upper, middle, lower trunks

Anterior divisions

Lateral cord

Medial cord

Lateral pectoral nerve

Medial pectoral nerve

Innervation

Innervation is via the medial and lateral pectoral nerves; medial and lateral cords; upper, middle, and lower trunks; and roots C_5, C_6, C_7, C_8, and T_1.

Origin

The pectoralis minor originates at the outer surfaces of the third to fifth ribs (frequently second to fourth).

Insertion

Insertion is at the coracoid process of the scapula.

Activation Maneuver

Depression of the shoulder activates the muscle.

EMG Needle Insertion

Insert the needle in the midclavicular line overlying the third rib.

Pitfalls

If the needle is inserted too superficially, it will be in the pectoralis major.

Clinical Comments

An isolated lesion of the lateral or medial pectoral nerves is rare.

Weakness of the pectoralis minor is unlikely to be clinically detectable.

Neurogenic EMG changes in the pectoralis minor may be seen with radiculopathies affecting the C_5–T_1 roots. This muscle is therefore of little benefit in localizing a root lesion.

In prolonged hyperabduction of the arm, the neurovascular bundle in the axilla can be stretched under the pectoralis minor tendon, resulting in symptoms of neurovascular compression (Pecina et al., 1997).

Cervical

Plexus

C_1

C_2

To deep muscles of
the neck

C_3

C_4

To levator scapulae

C_5

Join Spinal
Accessory Nerve — To sternocleidomastoid —

To trapezius —

Phrenic Nerve
to diaphragm

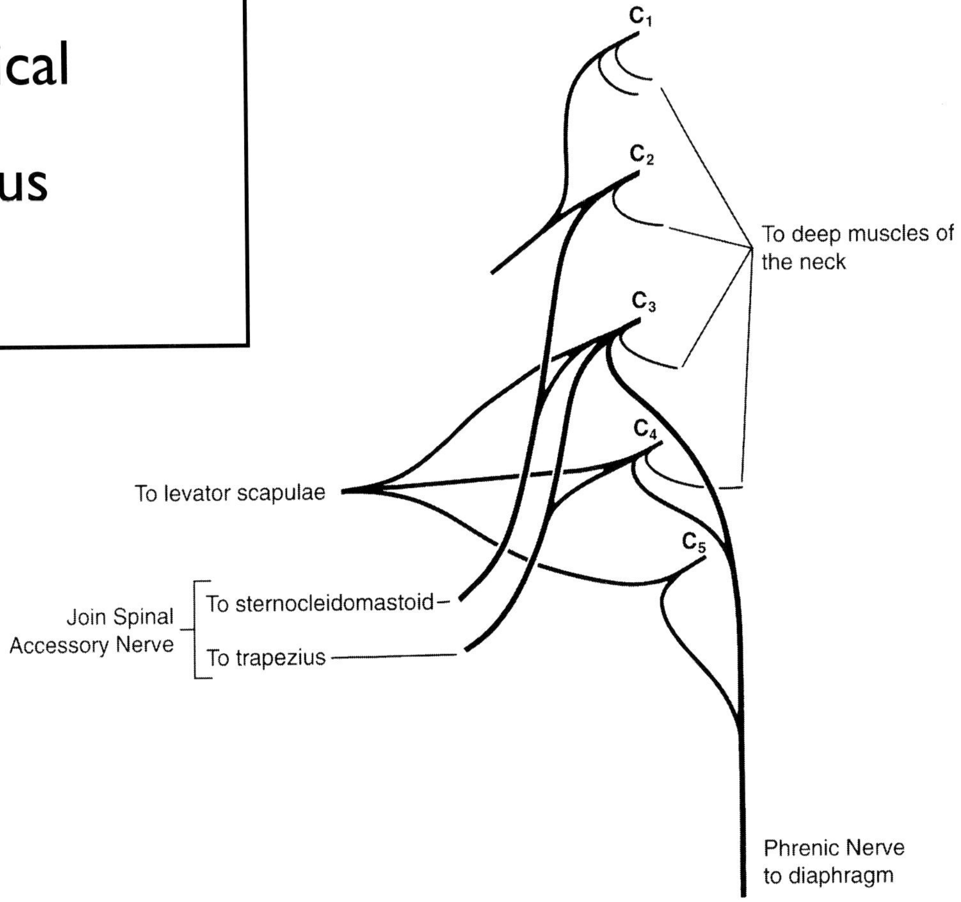

Diagram of the major muscular branches of the
cervical plexus (lateral view).

The cervical plexus is formed by the upper four
cervical ventral rami (Gray's Anatomy, 1977). It lies
deep to the sternocleidomastoid muscle and anterior to the scalenus medius and levator scapulae
muscles. Its branches can be divided into two
groups, *superficial* and *deep*. The superficial
branches provide cutaneous innervation to the
head, neck, and chest and include the lesser occipital, great auricular, transverse cervical, and supra-
clavicular nerves. The deep branches are largely
muscular branches distributed to deep muscles of
the neck, including the anterior recti and rectus
capitis lateralis muscles and the scalenus medius.
These branches also supply the sternocleidomastoid, trapezius, levator scapulae, and the diaphragm.

The diaphragm receives its motor supply solely

from the cervical plexus via the *phrenic nerve,* which arises from the third, fourth, and fifth cervical nerves. The muscular branches from the cervical plexus to the sternocleidomastoid and trapezius communicate with the *spinal accessory nerve,* which provides most of the innervation to these muscles. Cervical branches to the sternocleidomastoid are derived chiefly from the second and third cervical nerves, while branches to the trapezius are derived from the third and fourth cervical nerves. Branches to the levator scapulae are derived from the third and fourth cervical nerves, which are joined by the fifth cervical nerve via the *dorsal scapular nerve* of the brachial plexus.

REFERENCES

Berry H, MacDonald E A, Mrazek A C: Accessory nerve palsy: A review of 23 cases. Can J Neurol Sci 1991;18:337–341.

Donner T, Kline D G: Extracranial spinal accessory nerve injury. Neurosurgery 1993;32:907–911.

Gray's Anatomy. 15th English Edition. Bounty Books/Crown Publishers, New York, 1977, pp 758–764.

Gray's Anatomy. 38th Edition. Churchill Livingstone, New York, 1995, pp 1263–1266.

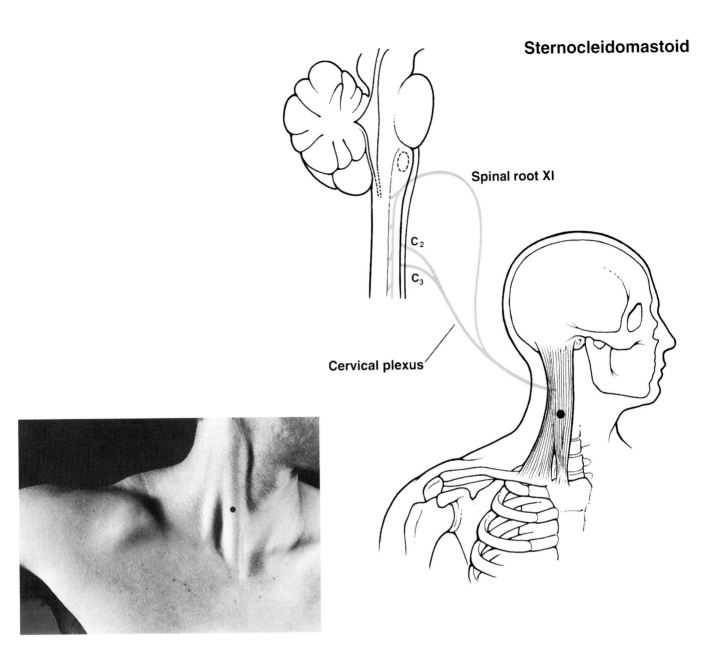

Spinal root XI

C_2

C_3

Cervical plexus

Innervation

Innervation is via the spinal accessory nerve and branches from the C_2, C_3, and sometimes the C_4 cervical spinal nerves (Gray's Anatomy, 1995).

Origin

The sternal head arises from the upper part of the manubrium sterni.

The clavicular head arises from the medial third of the clavicle.

Insertion

Insertion is at the lateral surface of the mastoid process.

Activation Maneuver

Rotation of the head (opposite to the muscle studied) activates the muscle.

EMG Needle Insertion

Insert the needle at the midpoint between the mastoid process and the sternal origin. Enter the muscle obliquely, and direct the needle parallel to the muscle fibers.

Pitfalls

If the needle is inserted too medially and anteriorly, it may penetrate the common, internal, or external carotid arteries.

Clinical Comments

Needle examination may show neurogenic changes when injury to the spinal accessory nerve or branches from C_2, C_3, and C_4 produces axonal loss. Note: The spinal accessory nerve may be damaged during lymph node dissection in the posterior triangle of the neck, sparing the sternocleidomastoid but affecting the trapezius (Donner and Kline, 1993).

Cervical dystonia (torticollis) often begins with tonic or clonic spasms of the sternocleidomastoid muscle.

Trapezius

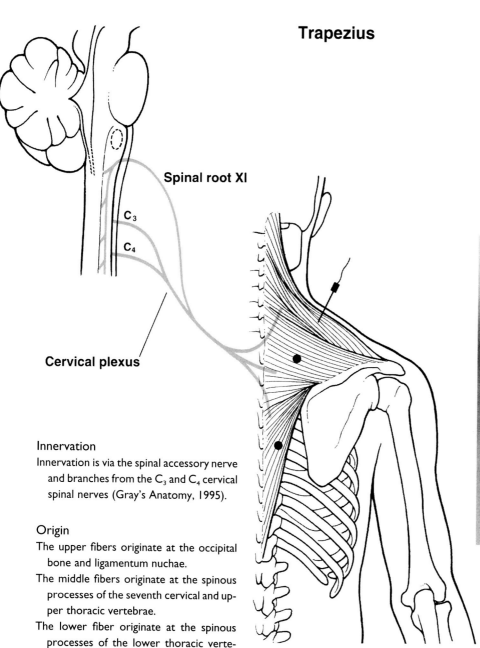

Spinal root XI

C₃

C₄

Cervical plexus

Innervation

Innervation is via the spinal accessory nerve and branches from the C_3 and C_4 cervical spinal nerves (Gray's Anatomy, 1995).

Origin

The upper fibers originate at the occipital bone and ligamentum nuchae.

The middle fibers originate at the spinous processes of the seventh cervical and upper thoracic vertebrae.

The lower fiber originate at the spinous processes of the lower thoracic vertebrae.

Insertion

Upper fibers: Insertion is at the outer third of posterior border of clavicle.

Middle fibers: Insertion is at the acromion process and the crest of the spine of the scapula.

Lower fibers: Insertion is at the medial surface of the spine of the scapula.

Activation Maneuver

Upper fibers: Shrug or elevate the shoulder.

Middle fibers: Retract the scapula.

Lower fibers: Rotate the scapula by elevating the arm.

EMG Needle Insertion

Upper fibers: Insert the needle at the angle of the neck and shoulder.

Middle fibers: Insert the needle midway between the spine of the scapula and the spinous processes at the same level.

Lower fibers: Insert the needle 3–4 cm lateral to the spinous processes of the lower thoracic vertebrae.

Pitfalls

Upper fibers: If the needle is inserted too deeply, it may be in the levator scapulae (supplied by the dorsal scapular nerve and C_3, C_4) or other neck muscles.

Middle fibers: If the needle is inserted too deeply, it may be in the rhomboideus major or minor, which are supplied by the dorsal scapular nerve.

Lower fibers: If the needle is inserted too deeply and caudally, it may be in the latissimus dorsi, which is supplied by the thoracodorsal nerve.

Clinical Comments

Needle examination may show neurogenic changes when injury to the spinal accessory nerve or branches from C_3 and C_4 produces axonal loss.

The most common etiology of spinal accessory mononeuropathy is iatrogenic injury related to biopsy of cervical lymph nodes in the posterior triangle of the neck or benign tumor removal (Berry et al., 1991; Donner and Kline, 1993). This type of injury affects the trapezius but spares the sternocleidomastoid.

Levator Scapulae

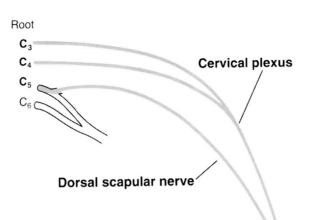

Root
C₃
C₄
C₅
C₆

Cervical plexus

Dorsal scapular nerve

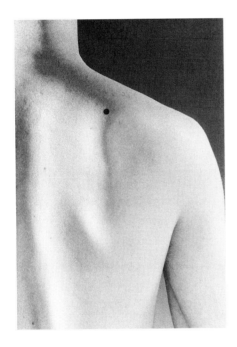

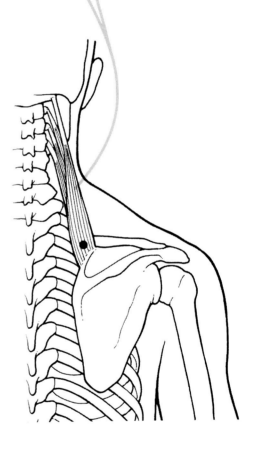

Innervation
Innervation is via the anterior rami of C₃, C₄, and C₅ and the latter branch via the dorsal scapular nerve.

Origin
The levator scapulae originate at the transverse processes of the upper four cervical vertebrae.

Insertion
Insertion is at the posteromedial border of the scapula, between the superior angle and the spine of the scapula.

Activation Maneuver
Elevation of the scapula (which assists the trapezius in the shrugging shoulders) activates the levator scapulae.

EMG Needle Insertion
Insert the needle along the superiomedial margin of the scapula.

Pitfalls
If the needle is inserted too superficially, it will be in the trapezius muscle, which is supplied by the spinal accessory nerve.

If the needle is inserted too deeply, it may be in the paraspinal muscles.

Clinical Comments
Neurogenic changes in this muscle on needle examination usually indicate C₃–C₅ radiculopathy.

Look for neurogenic changes in other C₅-innervated muscles to confirm C₅ radiculopathy.

Phrenic

Nerve

The phrenic nerve arises chiefly from the third and fourth cervical nerves, with a communicating branch from the fifth (Gray's Anatomy, 1977). It descends to the root of the neck beneath the sternocleidomastoid, the posterior belly of the omohyoid, and the transversalis colli muscles. It passes over the first part of the subclavian artery, lying between it and the subclavian vein. Within the chest the phrenic nerve descends almost vertically in front of the root of the lung and by the side of the pericardium, between it and the mediastinal portion of the pleura. It reaches the diaphragm, where it divides into branches that separately pierce the muscle and are distributed to its undersurface.

The two phrenic nerves differ in their length and in their anatomical relations in the upper thorax. The *right nerve* is shorter, more deeply situated, and more vertical in its descent than the left. It lies on the outer side of the right brachiocephalic vein and superior vena cave. The *left nerve* is longer due to the inclination of the heart to the left and from the diaphragm being lower on this side. It enters the thorax behind the left brachiocephalic vein and crosses in front of the vagus nerve, aortic arch, and root of the lung. In the thorax, each phrenic nerve is accompanied by a branch of the internal mammary artery.

PHRENIC NERVE LESION

Etiology

Trauma to the side of the neck causes direct nerve injury.

Iatrogenic causes include surgery in the neck, compression by retractors or other instruments, and subclavian vein catheterization (Drachler et al., 1976).

Neuralgic amyotrophy is causative.

Malignant neoplasms, including bronchogenic carcinoma and other lesions within the chest, can cause a phrenic nerve lesion.

Abnormalities may occur in C_3–C_5 radiculopathy, spinal cord injury or other pathological conditions affecting the anterior horn cells at the C_3–C_5 segments, motor neuron disease, and polyneuropathy.

General Comments

Lower motor neuron damage to the phrenic nerve may occur anywhere along its course, from the anterior horn cells at the C_3–C_5 segments to the terminal innervation of the diaphragm (Bolton, 1993).

Clinical Features

Dyspnea occurs. If there is incomplete injury to the high cervical cord, all respiratory movements will be weak and breathing will be rapid and shallow.

Weakness of diaphragm typically causes paradoxic respiration.

Electrodiagnostic Strategy

Perform phrenic nerve conduction studies (Bolton, 1993). In axonal loss lesions affecting the phrenic nerve, compound muscle action potentials from the diaphragm will be reduced or absent. In demyelinating lesions, phrenic nerve conduction latencies may be markedly prolonged.

Demonstrate neurogenic EMG changes in the diaphragm.

Evaluate for C_3, C_4, or C_5 radiculopathy by performing EMG in other muscles that have C_3–C_5 innervation (cervical paraspinals, sternocleidomastoid, trapezius, levator scapulae, and rhomboids).

Perform nerve conduction studies to assess for cervical or brachial plexus lesions.

REFERENCES

Bolton C F: AAEM minimonograph #40: Clinical neurophysiology of the respiratory system. Muscle Nerve 1993;16:809–818.

Bolton C F, Grand'Maison F, Parkes A, Shkrum M: Needle electromyography of the diaphragm. Muscle Nerve 1992;15:678–681.

Drachler D H, Koepke G H, Weg J G: Phrenic nerve injury from subclavian vein catheterization: Diagnosis by electromyography. JAMA 1976;236:2880–2881.

Gray's Anatomy. 15th English Edition. Bounty Books/Crown Publishers, New York, 1977, pp 758–764.

Diaphragm

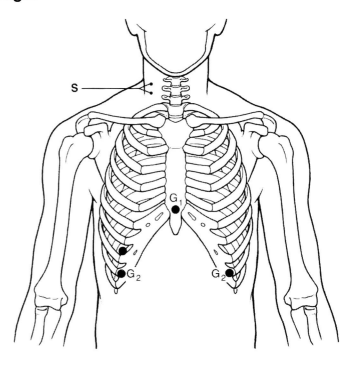

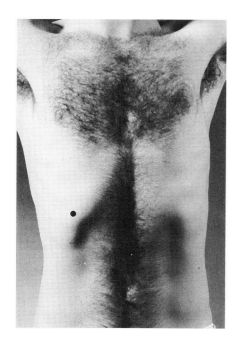

The techniques of phrenic nerve conduction and needle EMG of the chest wall and diaphragm. The phrenic nerve is stimulated (S) at the posterior border of the sternocleidomastoid muscle. The diaphragm compound muscle action potential is recorded from ipsilateral surface electrodes (G_1 and G_2). Needle EMG is recorded with the needle inserted at right angles to the chest wall in any one of several interspaces (in this example, the seventh and eighth rib interspace) between the anterior axillary and medial clavicular lines. There is at least 1.5 cm between the pleura above and the lower costal margin below, upon which the diaphragm inserts. Bursts of motor unit potentials characteristically occur with each inspiration when the needle is in the diaphragm. (From Bolton [1993], with permission.)

Innervation

Innervation is via the anterior rami of C_3, C_4, and C_5 via the cervical plexus ("C_3, C_4, C_5 keeps the diaphragm alive").

Origin

The diaphragm originates at the circumference of the thoracic cavity. The diaphragm separates the thorax from the abdomen.

Insertion

Anteriorly and laterally: Insertion is to the inner surface of the xiphoid cartilage and cartilages and bony portions of the six or seven inferior ribs.

Posteriorly: Insertion is to the aponeurotic arches and crura that attach to the lumbar vertebrae.

Activation Maneuver

There is activation of the diaphragm with each inspiration. Motor unit potentials (MUPs) in the diaphragm are of shorter duration and smaller amplitude, but are more numerous than MUPs from chest wall muscles (the needle will first pass through the external oblique or rectus abdominus muscles and the external and internal intercostal muscles before entering the diaphragm). With quiet respiration, the chest wall muscles do not fire or only recruit a few MUPs (Bolton, 1993).

EMG Needle Insertion

Introduce the needle at a right angle to the chest wall in any one of several interspaces (usually the seventh, eighth, or ninth rib interspace) between the anterior axillary and midclavicular lines. *The needle should be inserted just above the costal margin,* where there is an approximately 1.5-cm distance between the pleural reflection and the lower costal cartilage upon which the diaphragm inserts (see illustrations). Thus, the needle does not traverse either the pleural space or the lung.

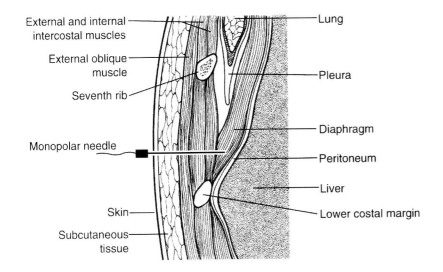

External and internal intercostal muscles

External oblique muscle

Seventh rib

Monopolar needle

Skin

Subcutaneous tissue

Lung

Pleura

Diaphragm

Peritoneum

Liver

Lower costal margin

Anatomy of needle EMG of the chest wall and diaphragm. The various structures that the needle traverses in reaching the diaphragm are shown. The distance between the cartilaginous lower costal margin and the pleural reflection is about 1.5 cm. In quiet respiration, the lung is well removed from the path of the needle. Entry of the needle into the peritoneum is associated with pain and loss of muscle insertional activity. (From Bolton [1993], with permission.)

Pitfalls

If the needle is inserted too deeply, it will enter the peritoneum. Entry of the needle into the peritoneum produces pain and loss of muscle insertional activity.

If the needle is inserted below the costal margin or at a more proximal interspace, it may penetrate the neurovascular bundle (intercostal nerve, artery, and vein) and continue into the pleura and lung.

Clinical Comments

The technique is reported to be safe, causes little discomfort, and provides good recordings of diaphragm activity (Bolton et al., 1992; Bolton, 1993).

Neurogenic changes, including abnormal spontaneous activity, can be recorded from chest wall muscles and diaphragm (Bolton, 1993).

If there is total denervation of the diaphragm, MUPs will not fire with attempted inspiration. Hence, an important sign that the needle is in the diaphragm will be lost.

Pneumothorax is a rare complication of this technique, particularly in patients with chronic obstructive pulmonary disease.

The phrenic nerve may be unilaterally damaged, as in radiculopathy, tumor, trauma, or surgery.

In high cervical spinal cord injury, denervation will usually be present in one or both diaphragms; MUPs will recruit in a neurogenic pattern or not at all if denervation is complete.

Look for neurogenic changes in other C_3–C_5 innervated muscles to support the diagnosis of radiculopathy or high cervical spinal cord injury. Muscles to be examined include cervical paraspinals, trapezius, levator scapulae, and rhomboids.

Sacral

Plexus

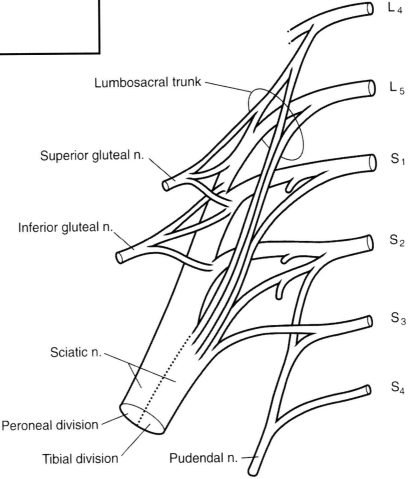

Diagram of the sacral plexus (anterior view) and its branches.

The sacral plexus is formed by the lumbosacral trunk (a small branch of the fourth lumbar ventral ramus that joins the fifth lumbar ventral ramus), the first through third sacral ventral rami, and part of the fourth ventral ramus (Gray's Anatomy, 1995). It adjoins the posterior pelvic wall anterior to the piriformis muscle and posterior to the internal iliac vessels, ureter, sigmoid colon, and terminal ileum.

Pelvic fascia separates the sacral plexus from the viscera of the pelvis. The upper rami proceed obliquely downward and outward, while the lower rami proceed nearly horizontally. All rami converge toward the greater sciatic foramen and unite to form two cords, an upper, larger one and a lower, smaller cord. The upper, larger cord is formed by the lumbosacral trunk (L_4, L_5) and the first (S_1), second (S_2), and part of the third (S_3) sacral ventral rami. This cord becomes the *sciatic nerve.* The lower, smaller cord is formed by portions of the second (S_2), third (S_3), and fourth (S_4) sacral ventral rami. This becomes the *pudendal nerve.* In addition, the sacral plexus can be divided into anterior and posterior divisions, with the tibial portion of the sciatic nerve formed by the anterior division and the peroneal portion formed by the posterior division.

Branches of the sacral plexus include muscular branches to the quadratus femoris and gemellus inferior (L_4, L_5, S_1), the obturator internus and gemellus superior (L_5, S_1, S_2), and the piriformis (S_1, S_2). Note the short muscles around the hip joint—quadratus femoris, gemellus superior, gemellus inferior, obturator internus, obturator externus (this muscle is supplied by the lumbar plexus via the obturator nerve), piriformis, and pectineus (this muscle is supplied by the lumbar plexus via the femoral nerve)—are largely innaccessible to direct observation. Because of the potential complications presented by their intimate relationship with important neurovascular structures, there is a total lack of EMG data in humans (Gray's Anatomy, 1995). Muscular branches also supply the levator ani, coccygeus, sphincter ani externus (S_4), and pelvic splanchnic nerves (S_2, S_3, S_4). The sacral plexus also gives rise to the *superior gluteal nerve* (L_4, L_5, S_1), which supplies the gluteus medius, gluteus minimus, and tensor fasciae latae; the *inferior gluteal nerve* (L_5, S_1, S_2) to the gluteus maximus; the posterior cutaneous nerve of the thigh (S_1, S_2, S_3); and the perforating cutaneous nerve (S_2, S_3).

A lesion of the sacral plexus produces a clinical picture similar to that seen with a sciatic nerve lesion, but with additional involvement of the gluteal muscles, tensor fasciae latae, and, occasionally, the anal sphincter.

SACRAL PLEXUS LESION

Etiology

Tumors and metastatic lesions can cause a sacral plexus lesion. Malignant infiltration is the most common cause of involvement of the lumbosacral plexus, usually due to spread of carcinoma of the cervix, uterus, prostate, or rectum (Gray's Anatomy, 1995).

Neuralgic amyotrophy (also known as *idiopathic lumbosacral plexopathy, acute idiopathic mononeuropathy,* or *lumbosacral plexus neuropathy;* Kimura, 1989) is causative.

Trauma, including pelvic fractures, stab wounds, or gunshot wounds, can cause a sacral plexus lesion.

Traction injury during orthopedic or other surgical manipulation (common during hip joint replacement) can cause a sacral plexus lesion.

Radiation plexopathy is causative.

Compression plexopathy occurs due to retroperitoneal hematomas, usually in hemophiliacs, in those with coagulopathies, or during anticoagulation therapy.

Compression lesions against the bony pelvis also occur and affect the common peroneal fibers maximally or exclusively. The greater vulnerability of the peroneal fibers is due, in part, to the more direct relationship of the posterior division, which comprises peroneal fibers, with the bony pelvis (Sunderland, 1968).

General Comments

Malignant infiltration usually gives rise to *painful* and slowly progressive paralysis unilaterally (Kimura, 1989).

Radiation plexopathy causes very slowly progressive, *painless* leg weakness, often bilateral.

Neuralgic amyotrophy is characterized by acute pain in one or both legs that precedes the onset of weakness and areflexia.

Clinical Features

The distribution of weakness is similar to that seen with a sciatic nerve lesion.

There can be additional weakness of the gluteal muscles, tensor fasciae latae, or anal sphincter.

Wasting of lower limb muscles occurs.

Numbness occurs over the posterior thigh, lateral half of the leg, and entire foot.

There is an absent or reduced Achille's stretch reflex.

Electrodiagnostic Strategy

Use nerve conduction studies to confirm a lesion involving the sacral plexus (low amplitude or unelicitable sensory responses from sural and superficial peroneal nerves and low amplitude or unelicitable motor responses from tibial and peroneal nerves). Sensory responses are normal in radiculopathies because the lesion is proximal to the dorsal root ganglion (preganglionic lesion) and the cell bodies in the ganglion maintain viability of the peripheral sensory fiber.

Demonstrate neurogenic EMG needle examination (i.e., spontaneous activity, abnormal motor unit potentials, and abnormal recruitment) in muscles supplied by the sacral plexus.

Use needle EMG to exclude lumbosacral radiculopathies. Radiculopathies produce neurogenic findings in paraspinal muscles as well as in limb muscles; plexopathies never do so because the plexus is formed by *ventral rami*, whereas paraspinal muscles are innervated by *posterior rami* (Wilbourn, 1985).

REFERENCES

Gray's Anatomy. 38th Edition. Churchill Livingstone, New York, 1995, pp 1282–1288.

Kimura J: Electrodiagnosis in Diseases of Nerve and Muscle. 2nd Edition. F A Davis, Philadelphia, 1989, pp 456–457.

Sunderland S: Nerves and Nerve Injuries. Williams & Wilkins, Baltimore, 1968, pp 1069–1095.

Wilbourn A J: Electrodiagnosis of plexopathies. Neurol Clin 1985;3: 511–529.

chapter

15

Sciatic

Nerve

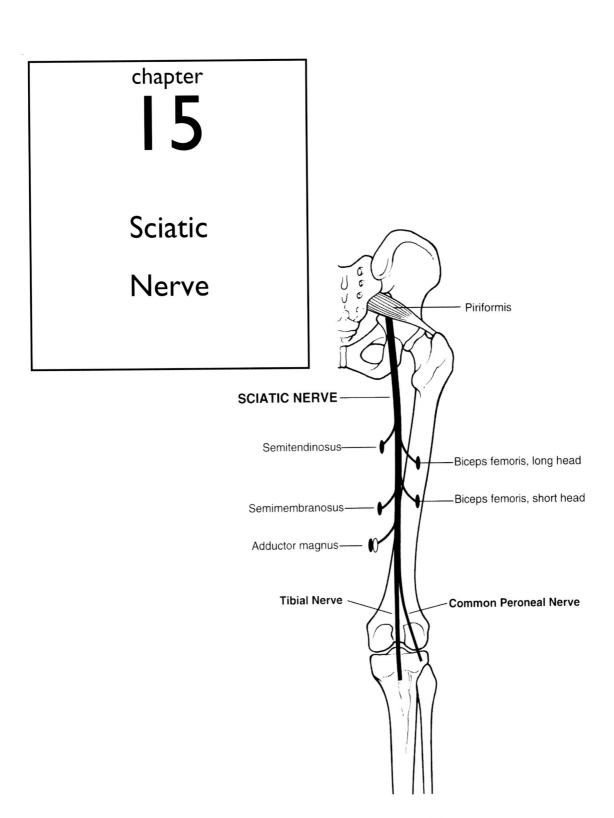

Piriformis

SCIATIC NERVE

Semitendinosus

Biceps femoris, long head

Biceps femoris, short head

Semimembranosus

Adductor magnus

Tibial Nerve

Common Peroneal Nerve

Diagram of the sciatic nerve (posterior view) and its branches. NOTE: The white oval signifies that a muscle receives part of its innervation from another peripheral nerve.

The sciatic nerve is a continuation of the upper, larger cord of the sacral plexus and is formed by the lumbosacral trunk (L_4, L_5) and the first, second, and part of the third sacral ventral rami (Gray's Anatomy, 1995). It is the broadest nerve of the human body (2 cm at its origin) and is composed of independent tibial and common peroneal divisions that are usually united as far as the lower part of the thigh, although simple dissection reveals the double structure. In about 10% of cases, the two divisions remain distinct from the outset. The sciatic nerve leaves the pelvis via the greater sciatic foramen below the lower margin of the *piriformis* muscle and descends between the greater trochanter of the femur and ischial tuberosity along the back of the thigh. Just above the popliteal fossa it separates into its two terminal divisions.

In the gluteal region (after emerging below the piriformis), the nerve is deep to the gluteus maximus. On leaving the gluteal region, the nerve continues down the midline of the thigh closely related to the shaft of the femur. Muscular branches are given to the biceps femoris (the short head is supplied by peroneal division and the long head by tibial division), semitendinosus, semimembranosus, and the ischiocondylar part of the adductor magnus. Articular branches supply the hip joint.

Although the sciatic nerve, or its branches, may be involved by penetrating injuries at any level, there are regions where the nerve is prone to certain types of injury. Anatomical features of particular clinical significance are found in the pelvis (see Chapter 14), the gluteal region, and the thigh (Sunderland, 1968). On leaving the pelvis, the nerve may rarely be entrapped by the piriformis muscle (piriformis syndrome). In the gluteal region the sciatic nerve is at risk because the buttock is a common site for therapeutic injections. The nerve is also intimately related to the hip joint and may be involved with injuries to that joint. Damage may also occur during operations on the hip joint or femur. In the thigh, the nerve may be injured during fractures of the femur or compressed against the firm edge of a seat.

SCIATIC NERVE LESION

Etiology
Tumors and metastatic lesions can cause a sciatic nerve lesion.

Trauma, including hip fracture or dislocation, or more distal fractures of the femur can cause a sciatic nerve lesion.

A traction injury can occur during orthopedic or other surgical manipulation (common during hip joint replacement).

Radiation therapy (usually related to radiation plexopathy) is causative.

Compression injury can occur in the gluteal region. As the nerve appears from beneath the gluteus maximus, it is relatively superficial and may be compressed when seated on a firm surface. Common peroneal fibers are maximally or exclusively affected (Sunderland, 1968).

Entrapment by the piriformis muscle (piriformis syndrome) can cause a sciatic nerve lesion.

Intramuscular injections can cause a sciatic nerve lesion. The nerve may be damaged by the needle, by sclerosing or toxic agents, or later by scarring that follows the tissue reaction (Sunderland, 1968).

General Comments
Malignant infiltration usually involves the nerve roots contributing to the formation of the sciatic nerve in the pelvis. It gives rise to *painful* and slowly progressive paralysis unilaterally (Kimura, 1989).

Radiation injury causes very slowly progressive *painless* leg weakness.

There is a greater vulnerability of the common peroneal fibers to most injuries of the sciatic nerve. This may be related to various factors, including the more exposed position of the peroneal division in the thigh, and to the poorer blood supply (less nutrient arteries). In addition, the size, number, and disposition of the funiculi may predispose the peroneal division to injury because it is composed of fewer and larger bundles with less connective tissue than the tibial division. Peroneal fibers are also securely fixed at both the sciatic notch and the neck of the fibula and therefore subjected to greater stretch (Sunderland, 1968).

Clinical Features

Weakness or wasting involves the hamstring muscles as well as the muscles supplied by the common peroneal and tibial nerves.

Numbness occurs over the lateral half of the leg and the entire foot.

The Achilles stretch reflex is absent or reduced.

Electrodiagnostic Strategy

Use nerve conduction studies to confirm a lesion involving the tibial and common peroneal fibers (low amplitude or unelicitable sensory responses from sural and superficial peroneal nerves, low amplitude or unelicitable motor responses from tibial and peroneal nerves).

Demonstrate neurogenic EMG needle examination (i.e., spontaneous activity, abnormal motor unit potentials, and abnormal recruitment) in muscles supplied by the sciatic nerve (hamstrings) and muscles supplied by the common peroneal and tibial nerves.

Use needle EMG to exclude lumbosacral radiculopathies. Radiculopathies produce neurogenic findings in paraspinal muscles as well as in limb muscles; peripheral nerve injury never does so because the peripheral nerve is formed by the *ventral rami* whereas the paraspinal muscles are innervated by the *posterior rami* (Wilbourn, 1985).

REFERENCES

Gray's Anatomy. 38th Edition. Churchill Livingstone, New York, 1995, pp 1282–1288.

Kimura J: Electrodiagnosis in Diseases of Nerve and Muscle. 2nd Edition. F A Davis, Philadelphia, 1989, pp 456–457.

Sunderland S: Nerves and Nerve Injuries. Williams & Wilkins, Baltimore, 1968, pp 1069–1095.

Wilbourn A J: Electrodiagnosis of plexopathies. Neurol Clin 1985;3:511–529.

Wilbourn A J: AAEE case report #12: Common peroneal mononeuropathy at the fibular head. Muscle Nerve 1986;9:825–836.

Roots

L₄

L₅

S₁

S₂

S₃

S₄

**Sciatic nerve
(tibial division)**

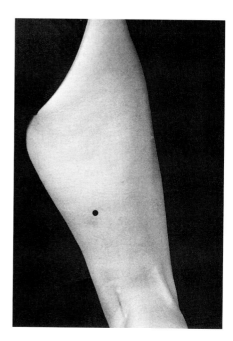

Innervation
Innervation is via the sciatic nerve (tibial division), sacral plexus, and roots. L_5, S_1, S_2.

Origin
The semitendinosus originates at the ischial tuberosity.

Insertion
Insertion is at the upper part of the medial surface of the shaft of the tibia.

Activation Maneuver
Flexion of the knee activates the muscle. Note: The "hamstrings" cross both hip and knee joints, integrating extension at the hip with flexion of the knee. In addition, the semitendinosus can act as a medial rotator of the leg.

EMG Needle Insertion
Insert the needle one-third to midway along a line connecting the semitendinosus tendon (easily palpable as it forms the proximal medial margin of the popliteal fossa) with the ischial tuberosity.

Pitfalls
There are no pitfalls. If the needle is inserted too laterally, it may be in the biceps femoris long head, which is also sup-

plied by the tibial division of sciatic nerve and roots L_5, S_1, and S_2. If the needle is inserted too medially, it may be in the semimembranosus (also the tibial division of the sciatic nerve and root L_5, S_1, S_2).

Clinical Comments
Neurogenic changes on needle examination may be seen with lesions of the tibial division of the sciatic nerve, sacral plexus, and roots L_5, S_1, or S_2.

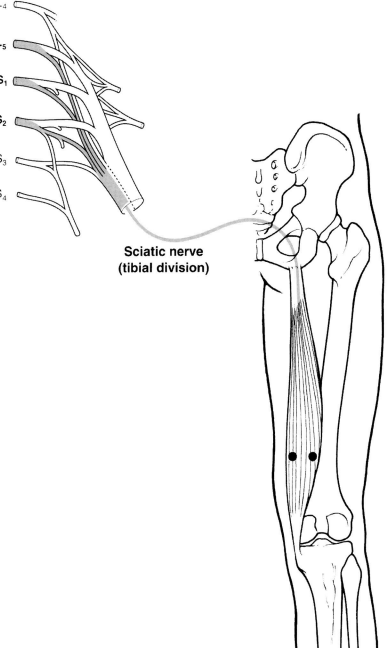

Sciatic nerve
(tibial division)

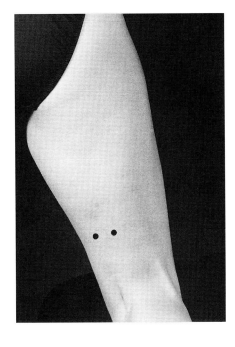

Innervation
Innervation is via the sciatic nerve (tibial division), sacral plexus, and roots L_5, S_1, S_2.

Origin
The semimembranosus originates at the ischial tuberosity.

Insertion
Insertion is at the medial condyle of the tibia (major insertion); it also inserts on the medial shaft of the tibia and the fascia over the popliteus and contributes to an expansion that inserts on the lateral femoral condyle.

Activation Maneuver
Flexion of the knee activates the muscle. Note: The "hamstrings" cross both hip and knee joints, integrating extension at the hip with flexion of the knee. In addition, the semimembranosus can act as a medial rotator of the leg.

EMG Needle Insertion
Palpate the semitendinosus tendon in the proximal popliteal fossa. Insert the needle on either side of the semitendinosus tendon.

Pitfalls
If the needle is inserted too laterally, it may be in the biceps femoris short head, which is supplied by the peroneal division of the sciatic nerve and roots L_5, S_1, S_2.
If the needle is inserted too medially and proximally, it may be in the adductor magnus or gracilis. The adductor magnus is supplied by the obturator nerve and the tibial division of the sciatic nerve (L_2–L_4 roots), while the gracilis receives innervation from the obturator nerve (L_2–L_3 roots).

Clinical Comments
Neurogenic changes on needle examination may be seen with lesions of the tibial division of the sciatic nerve, sacral plexus, and roots L_5, S_1 or S_2.

Roots

L₄

L₅

S₁

S₂

S₃

S₄

Biceps Femoris (Long Head)

Sciatic nerve
(tibial division)

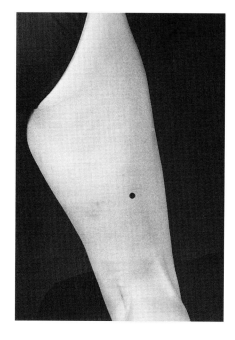

Innervation
Innervation is via the sciatic nerve (tibial division), sacral plexus, and roots L_5, S_1, S_2.

Origin
The long head of the biceps femoris originates at the ischial tuberosity.

Insertion
Insertion is at the head of the fibula.

Activation Maneuver
Flexion of the knee activates the muscle. Note: The "hamstrings" cross both hip and knee joints, integrating extension at the hip with flexion of the knee. In addition, the biceps femoris can act as a lateral rotator of the leg.

EMG Needle Insertion
Insert the needle one-third to midway along a line connecting the fibular head with the ischial tuberosity.

Pitfalls
If the needle is inserted too distally, it may be in the short head of the biceps femoris, which is supplied by the peroneal division of the sciatic nerve and roots L_5, S_1, S_2 (at the midthigh, the fibers of the short head are narrow and deep).

If the needle is inserted too laterally, it may be in the vastus lateralis, which is supplied by the femoral nerve (L_2–L_4 roots).

If the needle is inserted too medially, it may be in the semitendinosus, which is also supplied by the tibial division of the sciatic nerve (L_5–S_2 roots).

Clinical Comments
Neurogenic changes on needle examination may be seen with lesions of the tibial division of the sciatic nerve, sacral plexus, and roots L_5, S_1, or S_2.

Biceps Femoris (Short Head)

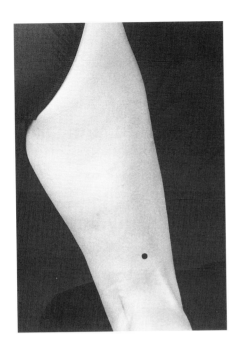

Roots
L₄
L₅
S₁
S₂
S₃
S₄

**Sciatic nerve
(peroneal division)**

Innervation
Innervation is via the sciatic nerve (peroneal division), sacral plexus, and roots L_5, S_1, S_2.

Origin
The short head of the biceps femoris originates at the lateral lip of the linea aspera on the posterolateral surface of the shaft of the femur and from the lateral intermuscular septum.

Insertion
Insertion is at the head of the fibula.

Activation Maneuver
Flexion of the knee activates the muscle. The short head of the biceps femoris does not cross the hip joint; it cannot contribute to hip extension, but it can act as a lateral rotator of the leg.

EMG Needle Insertion
Palpate the tendon of the long head of the biceps femoris in the popliteal fossa. Insert the needle just medial to the tendon.

Pitfalls
If the needle is inserted too laterally it may penetrate the long head of the biceps femoris, which is supplied by the tibial division of the sciatic nerve (roots L_5, S_1, S_2).

If the needle is inserted too medially, it may be in the semimembranosus, which is supplied by the tibial division of the sciatic nerve (roots L_5, S_1, S_2).

Clinical Comments
Neurogenic changes on needle examination may be seen with lesions of the peroneal division of the sciatic nerve, sacral plexus, and L_5, S_1, or S_2 roots.

This is the only muscle in the thigh innervated by the peroneal division of the sciatic nerve.

This muscle is of great importance in the electrodiagnostic evaluation of peroneal nerve lesions because it is crucial in defining the proximal extent of the lesion. If neurogenic EMG changes are present in this muscle, the lesion must be at or proximal to the midthigh (Wilbourn, 1986).

chapter
16

Tibial

Nerve

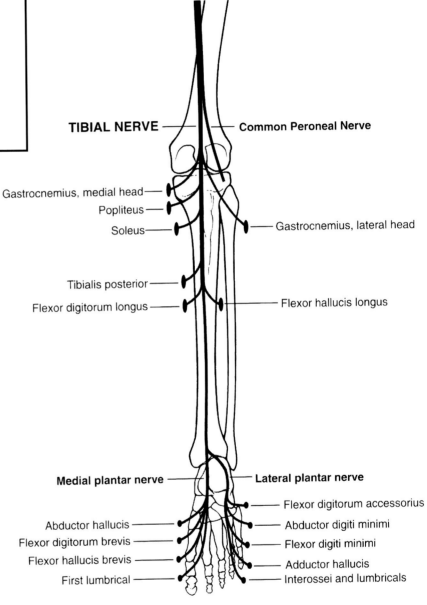

TIBIAL NERVE — **Common Peroneal Nerve**

Gastrocnemius, medial head
Popliteus
Soleus

Gastrocnemius, lateral head

Tibialis posterior
Flexor digitorum longus

Flexor hallucis longus

Medial plantar nerve — **Lateral plantar nerve**

Flexor digitorum accessorius
Abductor hallucis
Abductor digiti minimi
Flexor digitorum brevis
Flexor digiti minimi
Flexor hallucis brevis
Adductor hallucis
First lumbrical
Interossei and lumbricals

Diagram of the tibial nerve (posterior view) and
its branches.

The tibial nerve (also known as the *posterior tibial
nerve*) is the larger sciatic division and is formed by
the fourth and fifth lumbar and the first to third
sacral ventral rami (Gray's Anatomy, 1995). It descends along the back of the thigh and the popliteal
fossa to the distal border of the popliteus muscle,

passing anterior to the aponeurotic arch of the soleus with the popliteal artery and vein to enter the leg. In the distal thigh, it is overlapped by the hamstring muscles, but becomes more superficial in the popliteal fossa, where it is lateral to the popliteal vessels, becoming superficial to them at the knee and crossing to the medial side of the vessels as it enters the leg. In the distal fossa, it is overlapped by the junction of the two heads of the gastrocnemius muscles.

In the leg, the tibial nerve descends with the posterior tibial artery and vein, crossing lateral to the vessels. Proximally, the nerve is deep to the soleus and gastrocnemius, but in the distal one-third of the leg it is covered only by skin and fascia, sometimes overlapped by the flexor hallucis longus. It reaches the medial malleolus, ending under the flexor retinaculum, where it divides into medial and lateral plantar nerves.

The tibial nerve gives off articular branches to the knee joint. Just before it divides it also supplies the ankle joint. Most of the articular branches are nociceptive in nature. Muscular branches supply the two heads of the gastrocnemius, plantaris (a small, almost vestigial muscle that is the lower limb equivalent of the palmaris longus), soleus, popliteus, tibialis posterior, flexor digitorum longus, and flexor hallucis longus. Cutaneous branches include the sural and medial calcaneal nerves. The *sural nerve* is joined by a sural communicating branch of the common peroneal nerve and descends along the calf and lateral border of the Achilles tendon to the region between the lateral malleolus and the calcaneous. It supplies the posterior and lateral skin of the distal third of the leg, the skin overlying the lateral malleolus, and the lateral aspect of the foot and little toe (Sunderland, 1968). The medial calcaneal branch supplies the skin of the heel and the medial side of the sole.

The *medial plantar nerve* also gives off articular, cutaneous, and muscular branches. The cutaneous branches supply the skin of the sole of the foot, including the digital branches to the hallux, the second, third, and half of the fourth toe (the digital branches of the medial plantar nerve are like those of the median nerve). Muscular branches supply the abductor hallucis, flexor digitorum brevis, flexor hallucis brevis, and the first lumbrical (the muscular branches of the medial plantar nerve also correspond closely with those of the median nerve).

The *lateral plantar nerve* supplies the skin of the fifth toe, the lateral half of the fourth toe, and the lateral part of the sole of the foot (like the ulnar nerve in the hand). Muscular branches supply most deep muscles of the foot, including the flexor digitorum accessorius, abductor digiti minimi (quinti), flexor digiti minimi brevis, interossei, second to fourth lumbricals, and adductor hallucis.

The tibial nerve, or its branches, may be involved by penetrating injuries at any level. Of the two terminal divisions of the sciatic nerve, however, the tibial is the more deeply situated and better protected (Sunderland, 1968). At the ankle, the tibial nerve may rarely be subjected to compression beneath the flexor retinaculum (tarsal tunnel). This may result in the *tarsal tunnel syndrome*.

TARSAL TUNNEL SYNDROME

Etiology

Tarsal tunnel syndrome is caused by compression of the tibial nerve or its
  branches in the tarsal tunnel.

General Comments

Tarsal tunnel syndrome is a rare entrapment neuropathy.

Symptoms usually involve one foot (Dawson et al., 1990).

Predisposing conditions include trauma, such as fracture or dislocation at the
  ankle, deformity or hypermobility at the ankle, peripheral neuropathy,
  rheumatoid arthritis, and hyperlipidemia.

Radiologic studies of the ankle may reveal evidence of degenerative arthritis,
  old fractures, bone spicules, or accessory ossicals (DeLisa and Saeed,
  1983).

Clinical Features

Pain, reportedly burning in quality, occurs in the sole of the foot.

Patients may awaken at night with symptoms (nocturnal paresthesias).

Numbness may involve the medial plantar or lateral plantar areas and occasionally the whole surface of the foot, including the medial calcaneal
  distribution (Dawson et al., 1990).

Tinel's sign over the tarsal tunnel may be present (Oh et al., 1979).

Weakness and atrophy of the intrinsic foot muscles are difficult to detect
  clinically.

Electrodiagnostic Strategy

Use nerve conduction studies to confirm a focal lesion of the tibial sensory
  or motor fibers in the tarsal tunnel. Techniques have been developed for
  identifying conduction abnormalities within the tarsal tunnel (Oh et al.,
  1979; DeLisa and Saeed, 1983).

Perform EMG needle examination in the foot muscles innervated by both
  the medial and lateral plantar nerves. In tarsal tunnel syndrome associated
  with loss of motor fibers, EMG may show neurogenic changes (i.e., spontaneous activity, abnormal motor unit potentials, and abnormal recruitment).

If EMG examination of the foot muscles is abnormal, study the proximal
  tibial–innervated muscles to exclude a tibial nerve lesion above the ankle.
  Compare with the findings in the other foot because tarsal tunnel syndrome is often unilateral. Also, study the S_1 and S_2 muscles innervated by
  other nerves to exclude radiculopathy.

REFERENCES

Dawson D M, Hallett M, Millender L H: Entrapment Neuropathies. 2nd Edition. Little, Brown,
  Boston, 1990, pp 291–299.

DeLisa J A, Saeed M A: AAEE case report #8: The tarsal tunnel syndrome. Muscle Nerve 1983;6:664–670.

Gray's Anatomy. 38th Edition. Churchill Livingstone, New York, 1995, pp 1282–1288.

Oh S J, Sarala P K, Kuba T, Elmore R S: Tarsal tunnel syndrome: Electrophysiologic study. Ann Neurol 1979;5:327–330.

Sunderland S: Nerves and Nerve Injuries. Williams & Wilkins, Baltimore, 1968, pp 1069–1095.

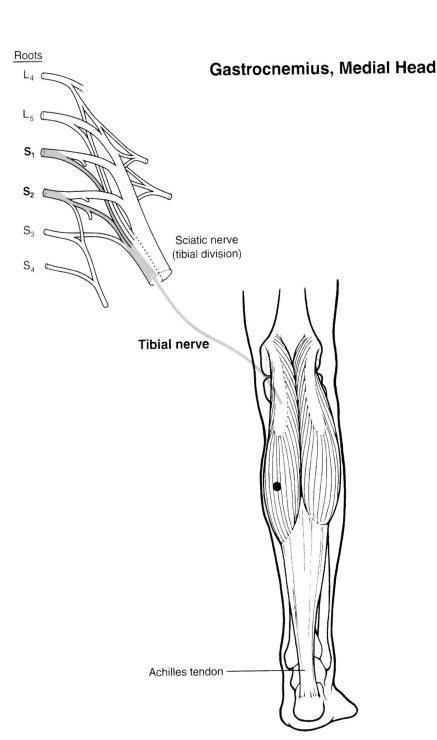

Roots
L₄
L₅
S₁
S₂
S₃
S₄

Sciatic nerve
(tibial division)

Gastrocnemius, Medial Head

Tibial nerve

Achilles tendon

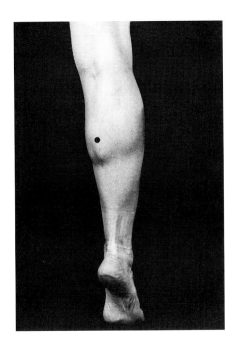

Innervation
Innervation is via the tibial nerve, tibial division of the sciatic nerve, sacral plexus, and roots S_1, S_2.

Origin
The medial head of the gastrocnemius originates at the medial condyle of the femur.

Insertion
Insertion is at the calcaneus via the Achilles tendon.

Activation Maneuver
Plantar flexion of the foot against resistance activates the muscle.

EMG Needle Insertion
Insert the needle into the medial mass of the calf.

Pitfalls
If the needle is inserted too deeply, it may be in the soleus, which is also supplied by the tibial nerve and S_1, S_2.

If the needle is inserted still deeper, it may be in the flexor digitorum longus or tibialis posterior (both muscles supplied by the tibial nerve and L_5, S_1). These muscles may show neurogenic changes on needle examination in an L_5 radiculopathy.

Clinical Comments
Neurogenic changes in the medial gastrocnemius on needle examination may be seen with lesions of the tibial nerve, sciatic nerve, sacral plexus, and S_1 or S_2 roots.

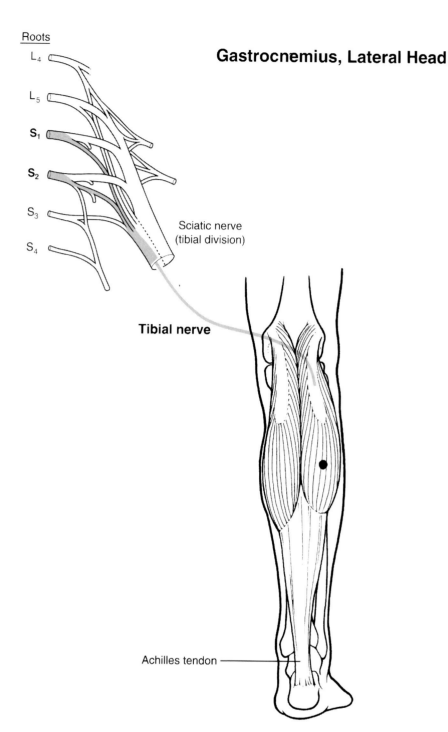

Gastrocnemius, Lateral Head

Roots
L₄
L₅
S₁
S₂
S₃
S₄

Sciatic nerve (tibial division)

Tibial nerve

Achilles tendon

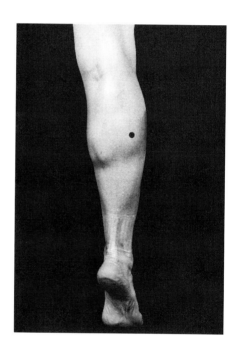

Innervation
Innervation is via the tibial nerve, tibial division of the sciatic nerve, sacral plexus, and roots S_1, S_2.

Origin
The lateral head of the gastrocnemius originates at the lateral condyle of the femur.

Insertion
Insertion is at the calcaneus via the Achilles tendon.

Activation Maneuver
Plantar flexion of the foot against resistance activates the muscle.

EMG Needle Insertion
Insert the needle into the lateral mass of the calf.

Pitfalls
If the needle is inserted too deeply, it may be in the soleus, which is also supplied by the tibial nerve and S_1, S_2.

If the needle is inserted too laterally and anteriorly, it may be in the peroneus longus or brevis, which are supplied by the superficial peroneal nerve. The outer border of the lateral gastrocnemius contacts the peronei muscles.

Clinical Comments
Neurogenic changes in this muscle on needle examination may be seen with lesions of the tibial nerve, sciatic nerve, sacral plexus, and S_1 or S_2 roots.

Soleus

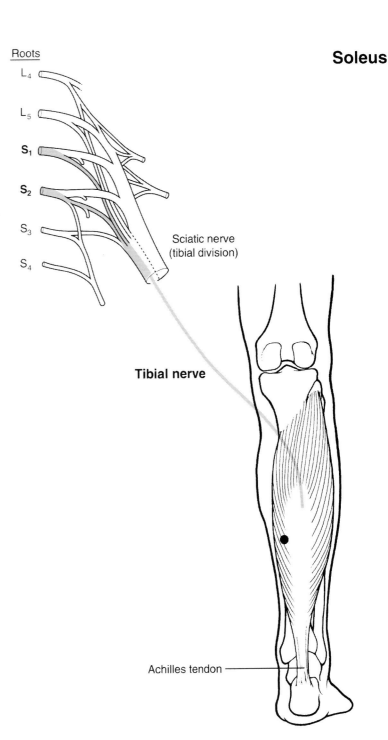

Roots

L₄
L₅
S₁
S₂
S₃
S₄

Sciatic nerve
(tibial division)

Tibial nerve

Achilles tendon

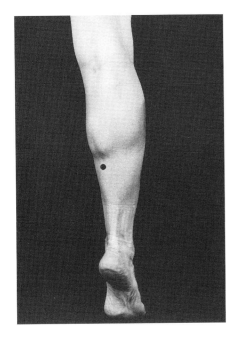

Innervation

Innervation is via the tibial nerve, tibial division of the sciatic nerve, sacral plexus, and roots S$_1$, S$_2$ (may also receive an L$_5$ contribution from the internal popliteal branch).

Origin

The soleus originates at the head of the fibula and the upper third of the posterior surface of its shaft and from the oblique line of the tibia and middle third of the medial surface of its shaft.

Insertion

Insertion is at the calcaneus via the Achilles tendon. Note: The Achilles tendon is the common tendon of the medial and lateral gastrocnemius and soleus muscles. These three muscles are sometimes referred to as the *triceps surae*.

Activation Maneuver

Plantar flexion of the foot against resistance activates the muscle.

EMG Needle Insertion

Insert the needle just distal to the belly of the medial gastrocnemius, medial to the Achilles tendon.

Pitfalls

If the needle is inserted too deeply, it may be in the flexor digitorum longus or tibialis posterior, which are supplied by the tibial nerve and L$_5$, S$_1$. These muscles may show neurogenic changes on needle examination in an L$_5$ radiculopathy.

Clinical Comments

Neurogenic changes in the soleus on needle examination may be seen with lesions of the tibial nerve, sciatic nerve, sacral plexus, and S$_1$ or S$_2$ roots. The soleus usually does not show neurogenic changes in an L$_5$ radiculopathy.

Tibialis Posterior

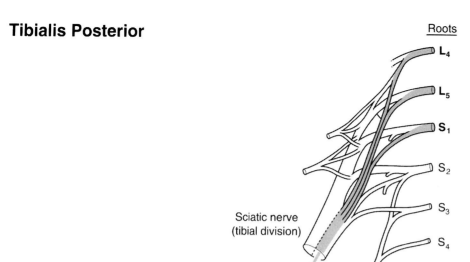

Roots

L₄

L₅

S₁

S₂

S₃

S₄

Sciatic nerve (tibial division)

Tibial nerve

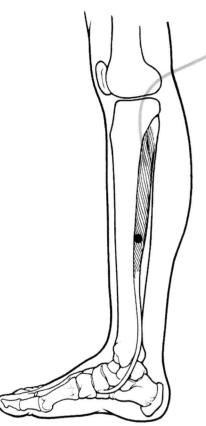

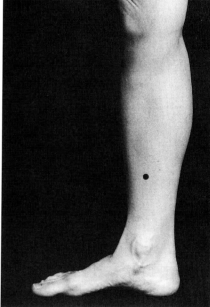

Innervation

Innervation is via the tibial nerve, tibial division of the sciatic nerve, sacral plexus, and roots L_5, S_1 (may also receive L_4 contribution).

Origin

The tibialis posterior originates at the posterior surface of the interosseous membrane throughout the entire length except at the lowest part, the posterior surface of the shaft of the tibia (between the oblique line and the junction of the middle and lower thirds of the shaft), and the upper two-thirds of the medial surface of the fibula.

Insertion

Insertion is at the tuberosity of the navicular and medial cuneiform bones (the tendon also gives off fibrous expansions to the sustentaculum tali of the calcaneus, middle and lateral cuneiform and cuboid bones, and bases of the second through fourth metatarsal bones).

Activation Maneuver

Inversion of the foot activates the muscle.

EMG Needle Insertion

Insert the needle 1–2 cm medial to the margin of the tibia at the junction of the upper two-thirds with the lower third of the shaft. Direct the needle obliquely (underneath the shaft) through the soleus and flexor digitorum muscles.

Pitfalls

If the needle is inserted too superficially, it will be in the flexor digitorum longus (also supplied by the tibial nerve and L_5, S_1) or soleus (supplied by the tibial nerve and S_1, S_2).

Clinical Comments

Neurogenic changes on needle examination may be seen with lesions of the tibial nerve, sciatic nerve, sacral plexus, and L_5, S_1 roots.

The tibialis posterior and flexor digitorum longus are usually abnormal in severe "foot drop" due to L_5 radiculopathy. Conversely, these muscles are normal in foot drop due to peroneal mononeuropathy.

Flexor Digitorum Longus

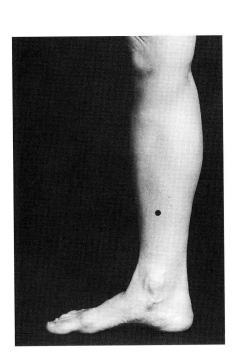

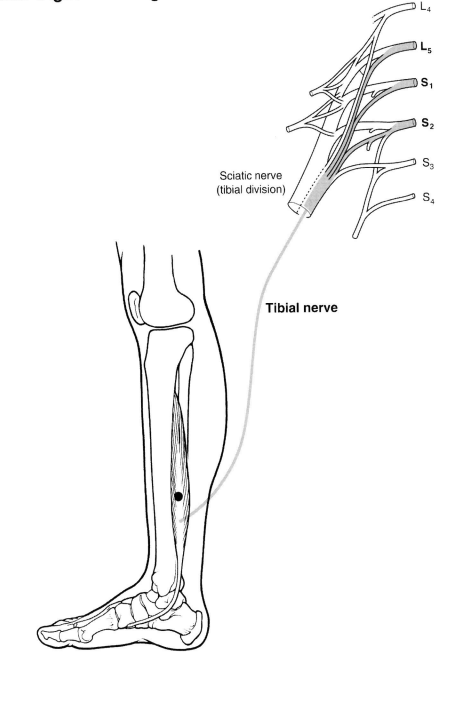

Sciatic nerve
(tibial division)

L$_4$

L$_5$

S$_1$

S$_2$

S$_3$

S$_4$

Tibial nerve

Innervation
Innervation is via the tibial nerve, tibial division of the sciatic nerve, sacral plexus, and roots L$_5$, S$_1$ (may also receive S$_2$ contribution).

Origin
The flexor digitorum longus originates at the posterior surface of the midshaft of the tibia immediately below the oblique line.

Insertion
Insertion is at the bases of the distal phalanges of the four lesser toes.

Activation Maneuver
Flexion of the four lesser toes without plantar flexion or inversion the foot (i.e., do not coactivate the soleus or tibialis posterior muscles) activates the muscle.

EMG Needle Insertion
Insert the needle 1–2 cm medial to the margin of the tibia at the junction of the upper two-thirds with the lower third of the shaft. Direct the needle obliquely (underneath the shaft) through the soleus muscle.

Pitfalls
If the needle is inserted too superficially, it will be in the soleus muscle (supplied by the tibial nerve and S$_1$, S$_2$).

If the needle is inserted too deeply, it will be in the tibialis posterior (also supplied by the tibial nerve and L$_5$, S$_1$).

Clinical Comments
Neurogenic changes on needle examination may be seen with lesions of the tibial nerve, sciatic nerve, sacral plexus, and L$_5$, S$_1$ roots.

The tibialis posterior and flexor digitorum longus are usually abnormal in severe "foot drop" due to L$_5$ radiculopathy. Conversely, these muscles are normal in foot drop due to peroneal mononeuropathy.

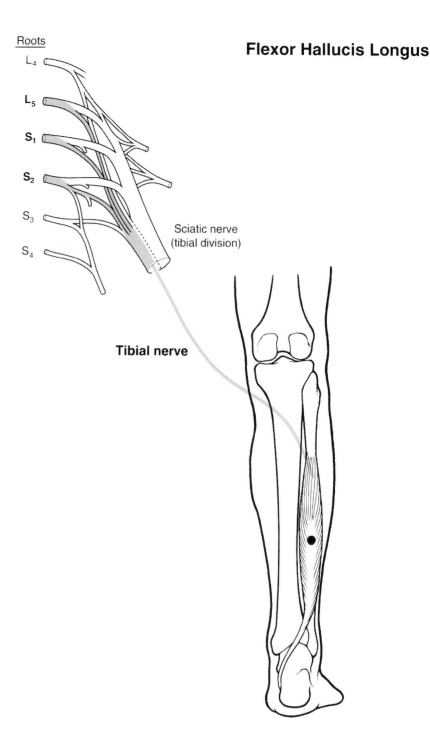

Flexor Hallucis Longus

Roots

L₄
L₅
S₁
S₂
S₃
S₄

Sciatic nerve
(tibial division)

Tibial nerve

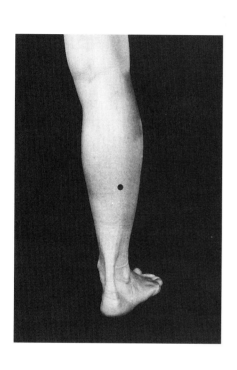

Innervation

Innervation is via the tibial nerve, tibial division of the sciatic nerve, sacral plexus, and roots L₅, S₁, S₂.

Origin

The flexor hallucis longus originates at the posterior surface of the distal two-thirds of the shaft of the fibula and the interosseous membrane.

Insertion

Insertion is at the base of the distal phalanx of the great toe.

Activation Maneuver

Flexion of the great toe without coactivation of other muscles activates the flexor hallucis longus.

EMG Needle Insertion

Insert the needle into the posterolateral aspect of the leg, at the junction of the upper two-thirds with the lower third. The muscle belly is situated deep on the fibular side of the leg and is larger than the flexor digitorum or tibialis posterior.

Pitfalls

If the needle is inserted too superficially, it will be in the soleus muscle (supplied by the tibial nerve and S₁, S₂).

If the needle is inserted too medially and deeply, it will be in the tibialis posterior (also supplied by the tibial nerve and L₅, S₁).

If the needle is inserted too laterally, it will be in the peroneus longus or brevis (supplied by the superficial peroneal nerve and L₅, S₁, S₂). The outer border of the flexor hallucis longus abuts the peronei muscles.

Clinical Comments

Neurogenic changes on needle examination may be seen with lesions of the tibial nerve, sciatic nerve, sacral plexus, and L₅, S₁, or S₂ roots.

Popliteus

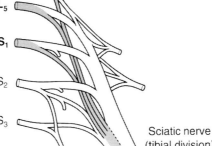

Roots

L$_4$

L$_5$

S$_1$

S$_2$

S$_3$

S$_4$

Sciatic nerve
(tibial division)

Tibial nerve

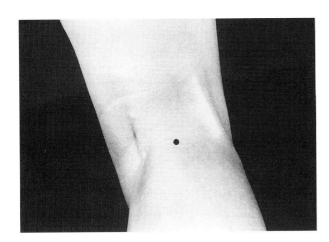

Innervation

Innervation is via the tibial nerve, tibial division of the sciatic nerve, the sacral plexus, and roots L$_4$, L$_5$, S$_1$.

Origin

The popliteus originates at the lateral condyle of the femur and the posterior ligament of the knee joint.

Insertion

Insertion is at the posterior surface of the shaft of the tibia above the oblique line.

Activation Maneuver

Flexion of the knee joint activates the muscle. (The popliteus produces a slight inward rotation of the tibia, which is es-

sential during the early stages of bending the knee.)

EMG Needle Insertion

Insert the needle into the floor of the popliteal fossa in the proximal leg midway between the insertions of the outer and inner hamstring tendons.

Pitfalls

Testing of the popliteus is rarely useful in routine electromyography due to the

muscle's thinness and proximity to the popliteal vessels.

If the needle is inserted too superficially, it will be in the gastrocnemius muscles (supplied by the tibial nerve and S$_1$, S$_2$).

Clinical Comments

Neurogenic changes on needle examination may be seen with lesions of the tibial nerve, sciatic nerve, sacral plexus, and roots L$_4$, L$_5$, or S$_1$.

Abductor Hallucis

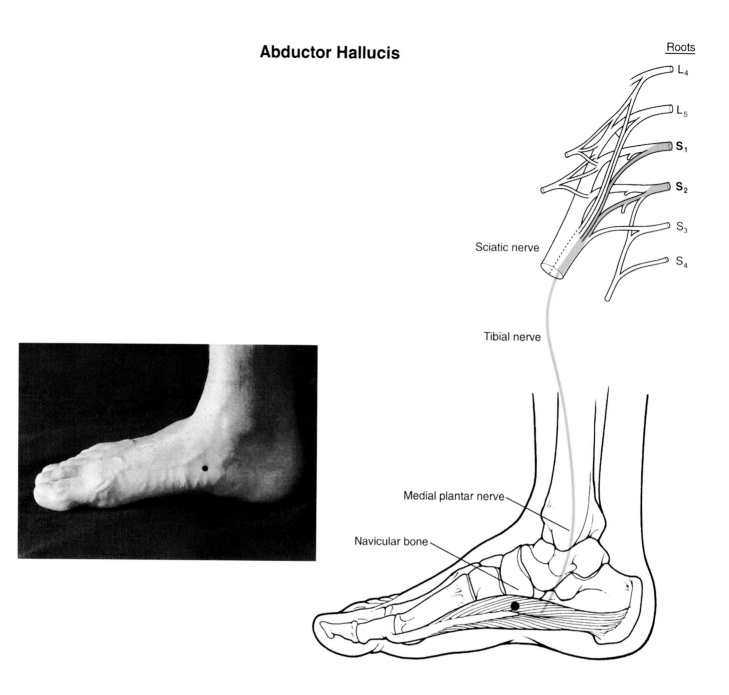

Roots

L₄

L₅

S₁

S₂

S₃

S₄

Sciatic nerve

Tibial nerve

Medial plantar nerve

Navicular bone

Innervation
Innervation is via the medial planter nerve, tibial nerve, tibial division of the sciatic nerve, sacral plexus, and roots S_1, S_2.

Origin
The abductor hallucis originates at the medial process of the calcaneus (heel bone).

Insertion
Insertion is at the base of the first phalanx of the great toe.

Activation Maneuver
Abduction of the great toe activates the muscle.

EMG Needle Insertion
Insert the needle into the muscle belly directly beneath the navicular bone.

Pitfalls
Some subjects may not be able to voluntarily activate this muscle.

If the needle is inserted too deeply, it may be in the flexor hallucis brevis muscle

(also supplied by the medial plantar nerve and S_1, S_2).

Clinical Comments
Neurogenic changes on needle examination may be seen with lesions of the medial plantar nerve, tibial nerve, sciatic nerve, sacral plexus, and S_1 or S_2 root.

The abductor hallucis is involved in the tarsal tunnel syndrome.

The abductor hallucis is also involved early in length-dependent peripheral neuropathies.

Flexor Digitorum Brevis

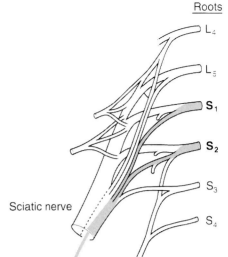

L₄
L₅
S₁
S₂
S₃
S₄

Sciatic nerve

Tibial nerve

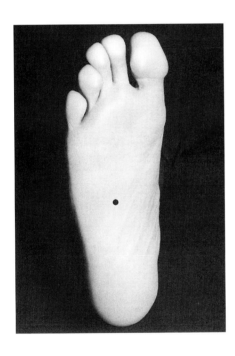

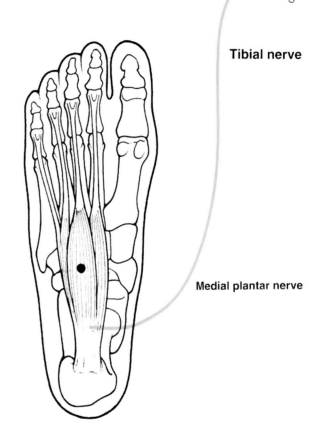

Medial plantar nerve

Innervation

Innervation is via the medial plantar nerve, tibial nerve, tibial division of the sciatic nerve, sacral plexus, and roots S_1, S_2.

Origin

The flexor digitorum brevis originates at the medial process of the calcaneus (heel bone) and the central part of the plantar aponeurosis.

Insertion

Insertion is at the bases of the middle phalanges of the second, third, fourth, and fifth toes.

Activation Maneuver

Flexion of the four lesser toes activates the muscle.

EMG Needle Insertion

Insert the needle midway between the third metatarsal head and the calcaneus. The muscle is superficial.

Pitfalls

If the needle is inserted too laterally, it may be in the abductor digiti minimi (quinti) or other muscles innervated by the lateral plantar nerve.

Clinical Comments

Neurogenic changes on needle examination may be seen with lesions of the medial plantar nerve, tibial nerve, sciatic nerve, sacral plexus, and S_1 or S_2 root.

The flexor digitorum brevis is involved in tarsal tunnel syndrome.

The flexor digitorum brevis is also involved early in length-dependent peripheral neuropathies.

TIBIAL NERVE   131

Flexor Hallucis Brevis

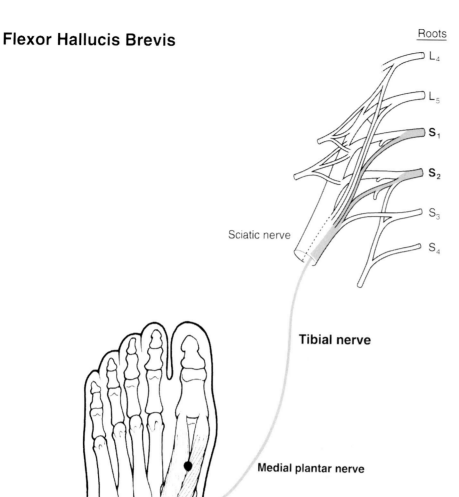

Roots
L₄
L₅
S₁
S₂
S₃
S₄

Sciatic nerve

Tibial nerve

Medial plantar nerve

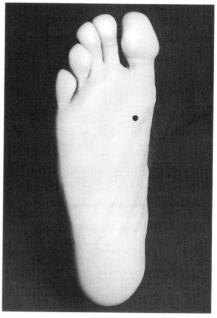

Innervation
Innervation is via the medial plantar nerve, tibial nerve, tibial division of the sciatic nerve, sacral plexus, and roots S_1, S_2.

Origin
The flexor hallucis brevis originates at the plantar surface of the cuboid, the lateral cuneiform, and the tendon of the tibialis posterior.

Insertion
Twin tendons attach to the base of the first phalanx of the great toe.

Activation Maneuver
Flexion of the great toe at the metatarsophalangeal joint activates the muscle.

EMG Needle Insertion
Insert the needle into the plantar surface of the foot 2 cm proximal to the first metatarsal head.

Pitfalls
If the needle is inserted too laterally, it may be in the adductor hallucis (supplied by the lateral plantar nerve and S_1, S_2, S_3).

The abductor hallucis is superficial to the flexor hallucis brevis, but it is also innervated by the medial plantar nerve and S_1, S_2.

Clinical Comments
Neurogenic changes on needle examination may be seen with lesions of the medial plantar nerve, tibial nerve, sciatic nerve, sacral plexus, and S_1 or S_2 root.

The flexor hallucis brevis is involved in the tarsal tunnel syndrome.

The flexor hallucis brevis is also involved early in length-dependent peripheral neuropathies.

Abductor Digiti Minimi (Quinti)

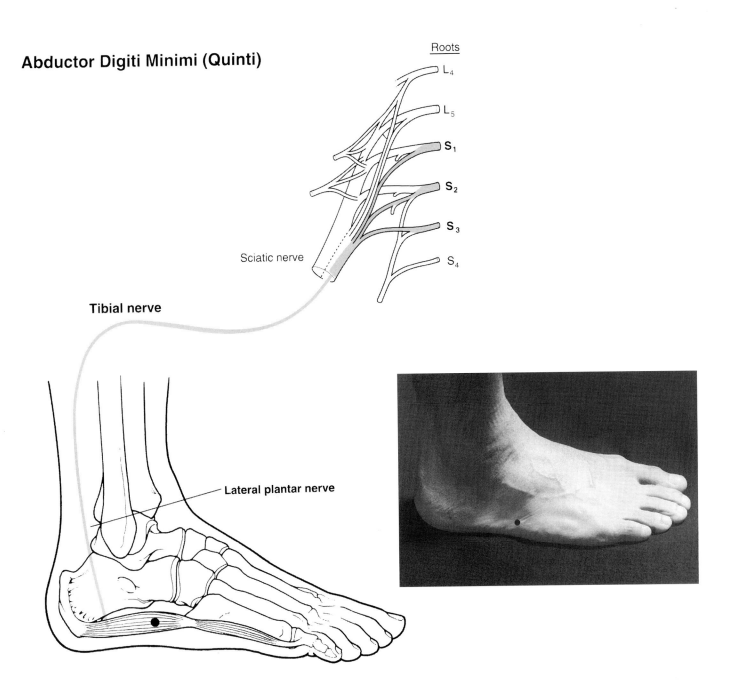

Roots

L₄

L₅

S₁

S₂

S₃

S₄

Sciatic nerve

Tibial nerve

Lateral plantar nerve

Innervation

Innervation is via the lateral plantar nerve, tibial nerve, tibial division of the sciatic nerve, sacral plexus, and roots S_1, S_2, S_3.

Origin

The abductor digiti minimi (quinti) originates at the medial and lateral processes of the calcaneus (heel bone) and the plantar aponeurosis. This muscle lies superficially along the lateral border of the foot.

Insertion

Insertion is at the lateral side of the base of the proximal phalanx of the fifth toe.

Activation Maneuver

Abduction or flexion of the fifth toe activates the muscle.

EMG Needle Insertion

Insert the needle along the lateral border of the foot midway between the fifth metatarsal head and the calcaneus.

Pitfalls

There are no pitfalls. If the needle is inserted too deeply, it will still be in muscles innervated by the lateral plantar nerve.

Clinical Comments

Neurogenic changes on needle examination may be seen with lesions of the lateral plantar nerve, tibial nerve, sciatic nerve, sacral plexus, and roots S_1, S_2, or S_3.

The abductor digiti minimi (quinti) is involved in the tarsal tunnel syndrome.

The abductor digiti minimi (quinti) is also involved early in length-dependent peripheral neuropathies.

Adductor Hallucis

Roots

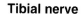

L₄
L₅
S₁
S₂
S₃
S₄

Sciatic nerve

Tibial nerve

Lateral plantar nerve

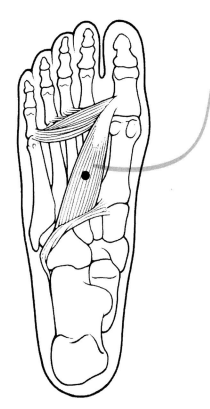

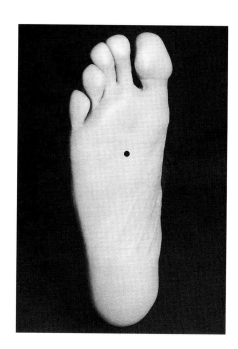

Innervation
Innervation is via the lateral plantar nerve, tibial nerve, tibial division of the sciatic nerve, sacral plexus, and roots S_1, S_2, S_3.

Origin
The oblique head originates from the bases of the second, third, and fourth metatarsal bones and from the fibrous sheath of the tendon of the peroneus longus.

The transverse head originates from the plantar metatarsophalangeal ligaments of the third, fourth, and fifth toes.

Insertion
Insertion is at the medial side of the base of the proximal phalanx of the great toe and the lateral sesamoid bone of the great toe.

Activation Maneuver
Adduction of the great toe activates the muscle.

EMG Needle Insertion
Insert the needle 4–5 cm proximal to the second metatarsal head to a depth of 2 cm or more (the muscle lies deep). This will access the thick, fleshy oblique head.

Pitfalls
If the needle is inserted too medially, it may be in the flexor hallucis brevis, which is innervated by the medial planter nerve.

If the needle is inserted too superficially, it may be in the first lumbrical, which is innervated by the medial plantar nerve.

Clinical Comments
Neurogenic changes on needle examination may be seen with lesions of the lateral plantar nerve, tibial nerve, sciatic nerve, sacral plexus, and roots S_1, S_2, or S_3.

The adductor hallucis is involved in the tarsal tunnel syndrome.

The adductor hallucis is also involved early in length-dependent peripheral neuropathies.

chapter
17

Common

Peroneal Nerve

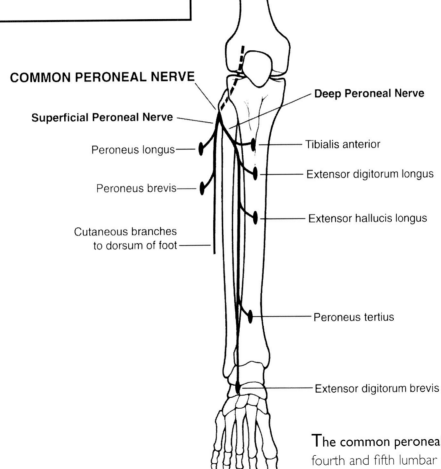

COMMON PERONEAL NERVE

Deep Peroneal Nerve

Superficial Peroneal Nerve

Peroneus longus

Tibialis anterior

Peroneus brevis

Extensor digitorum longus

Extensor hallucis longus

Cutaneous branches
to dorsum of foot

Peroneus tertius

Extensor digitorum brevis

Diagram of the common peroneal nerve (anterior view) and its branches.

The **common peroneal nerve** is derived from the fourth and fifth lumbar and first and second sacral ventral rami (Gray's Anatomy, 1995). It descends obliquely along the lateral side of the popliteal fossa, medial to the tendon of the biceps femoris as far as the attachment of the latter to the head of the fibula. It gives off two cutaneous branches, the lateral sural nerve (lateral cutaneous nerve of the calf) and the sural communicating nerve. The former supplies the skin of the anterior, lateral, and posterior aspects of the leg, the latter descends medially to join the sural nerve in the furrow between the two gastrocnemius muscles. Articular branches in the fossa supply the knee joint. The nerve then curves laterally around the neck of the fibula, passing between the two heads of the peroneus longus before dividing into its two terminal branches: the *superficial peroneal* and the *deep peroneal* nerves. At the neck of the fibula, the nerve is flattened and superficial and can be easily rolled against the bone (Sunderland, 1968).

The deep peroneal nerve (also known as the *anterior tibial nerve*) passes medially deep to the extensor digitorum longus and in front of the interosseous membrane. It descends on the interosseous membrane to the ankle, dividing there into lateral and medial terminal branches. Muscular branches in the leg supply the tibialis anterior, extensor digitorum longus, extensor hallucis longus, and peroneus tertius. The lateral terminal branch runs laterally on the dorsum of the foot to supply the extensor digitorum brevis. It also gives off interosseous branches to the tarsal and metatarsophalangeal joints and to the second dorsal interosseous muscle. The medial terminal branch runs distally on the dorsum of the foot and terminates in the first interspace where it provides cutaneous innervation to the skin on the contiguous sides of the great and second toes. It also gives off branches to the tarsal and metatarsophalangeal joints and the first dorsal interosseous muscle.

The superficial peroneal nerve turns downward between the peroneus longus and the extensor digitorum longus and emerges from between them at the mid to lower third of the leg, where it divides into lateral and medial terminal branches. In its course it supplies the peroneus longus and the peroneus brevis. The two terminal branches are cutaneous. The medial supplies the medial aspect of the dorsum of the foot, medial side of the great toe, and the contiguous sides of the second and third toes. The lateral supplies the lateral aspect of the dorsum of the foot and adjoining sides of the third and fourth, and fourth and fifth toes.

While the common peroneal nerve, or its branches, may be involved by penetrating injuries at any level, there are regions where the nerve is prone to certain types of injury. In the popliteal fossa, the nerve is intimately related to the knee joint as it curves laterally to reach the head of the fibula. In this position the nerve may be stretched or torn in medial (adduction) dislocations of the knee joint (Sunderland, 1968). At the head and neck of the fibula, the nerve is superficial and may be damaged by fractures of the fibula, blows to the lateral side of the knee, superficial lacerations, pressure from improperly applied casts, compression or ischemia resulting from habitual leg crossing, or compression against any hard surface. Emaciation and weight loss are also conditions that predispose the nerve to injury.

COMMON PERONEAL MONONEUROPATHY AT THE KNEE

Etiology
Injury to the common peroneal nerve or its branches as the nerve winds around the head and neck of the fibula can cause common peroneal mononeurophathy at the knee.

The condition is usually traumatic in origin due to compression, traction, or laceration.

General Comments
Mononeuropathy at the knee is common.

Compression can cause nerve dysfunction by both a single episode and by repeated episodes (e.g., habitual leg crossing).

Unilateral symptoms are more common, but bilateral asymmetrical involvement is often seen in patients who are habitual leg crossers, are emaciated and bedridden, or have sustained nerve infarcts from vasculitis (Wilbourn, 1986).

Clinical Features
There is weakness of foot dorsiflexion ("foot drop"). This is the chief complaint in almost all patients.

Weakness occurs during extension of the toes.

Weakness of foot eversion can occur (due to involvement of the superficial peroneal fibers that supply the peroneus longus and brevis). Note: foot eversion may be normal in some patients with common peroneal mononeuropathy at the knee.

Loss of sensation or numbness can occur over the anterolateral part of the leg and the dorsum of the foot.

Electrodiagnostic Strategy
Use nerve conduction studies to confirm a focal lesion of common peroneal motor and sensory fibers at the fibular head. Routine techniques are available that can identify conduction abnormalities across the fibular head (Katirji and Wilbourn, 1984; Wilbourn, 1986).

Perform EMG needle examination in muscles innervated by both the deep peroneal nerve and the superficial peroneal nerve. In common peroneal mononeuropathy associated with loss of motor fibers, EMG will show neurogenic changes (i.e., spontaneous activity, abnormal motor unit potentials, and abnormal recruitment).

If EMG is abnormal in muscles innervated by the common peroneal nerve, study the biceps femoris (short head) to define the proximal extent of the lesion (i.e., neurogenic changes in this muscle suggest a sciatic mononeuropathy with disproportionate involvement of common peroneal fibers).

Exclude L_5 radiculopathy as the etiology of foot drop (perform a needle examination in the tensor fasciae latae, gluteus medius, and lumbosacral paraspinal muscles).

REFERENCES

Dawson D M, Hallett M, Millender L H: Entrapment Neuropathies. 2nd Edition. Little, Brown, Boston, 1990, pp 295–299.

Gray's Anatomy. 38th Edition. Churchill Livingstone, New York, 1995, pp 1282–1288.

Gutmann L: AAEM Minimonograph #2: Important anomalous innervations of the extremities. Muscle Nerve 1993;16:339–347.

Katirji M B, Wilbourn A J: Common peroneal mononeuropathy: A clinical electrophysiological study of 100 cases. Neurology 1984;34:142.

Sunderland S: Nerves and Nerve Injuries. Williams & Wilkins, Baltimore, 1968, pp 1069–1095.

Wilbourn A J: AAEE case report #12: Common peroneal mononeuropathy at the fibular head. Muscle Nerve 1986;9:825–836.

Tibialis Anterior

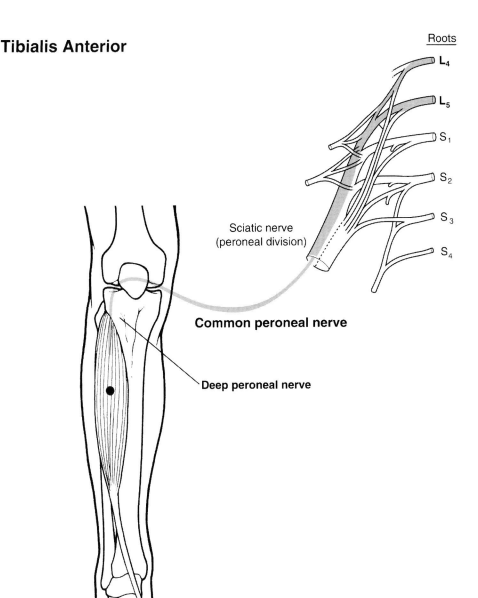

Roots

L$_4$

L$_5$

S$_1$

S$_2$

S$_3$

S$_4$

Sciatic nerve
(peroneal division)

Common peroneal nerve

Deep peroneal nerve

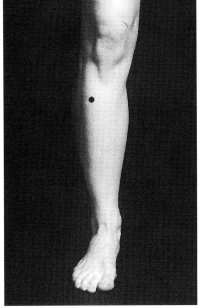

Innervation

Innervation is via the deep peroneal nerve, common peroneal nerve, peroneal division of the sciatic nerve, sacral plexus, and roots L$_4$, L$_5$.

Origin

The tibialis anterior originates from the lateral condyle of the tibia and the proximal half of the lateral surface of the shaft of the tibia.

Insertion

Insertion is at the medial cuneiform bone and adjoining part of the base of the first metatarsal bone.

Activation Maneuver

Dorsiflexion of the foot activates the muscle.

EMG Needle Insertion

Insert the needle just lateral to the proximal half of the shaft of the tibia (the muscle is superficial and readily palpable lateral to the tibia).

Pitfalls

There are no pitfalls. If the needle is inserted too laterally or deeply, it will be in the extensor digitorum longus, which is also innervated by the deep peroneal nerve.

Clinical Comments

Neurogenic changes on needle examination may be seen with lesions of the deep peroneal nerve, common peroneal nerve, peroneal division of the sciatic nerve, sacral plexus, or L$_4$, L$_5$ roots.

In the evaluation of severe "foot drop," always examine L$_5$ muscles that are *not* supplied by the common peroneal nerve (i.e., tibialis posterior, flexor digitorum longus, tensor fasciae latae, gluteus medius, or paraspinals) to exclude an L$_5$ radiculopathy. Conversely, these muscles are normal in foot drop due solely to peroneal mononeuropathy.

The tibialis anterior may also contribute to *inversion* of the foot because its tendon inserts on the medial aspect of the foot.

Extensor Digitorum Longus

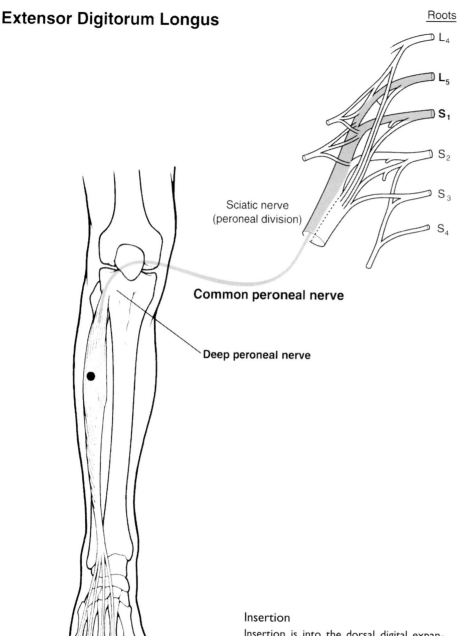

Roots

L₄

L₅

S₁

S₂

S₃

S₄

Sciatic nerve
(peroneal division)

Common peroneal nerve

Deep peroneal nerve

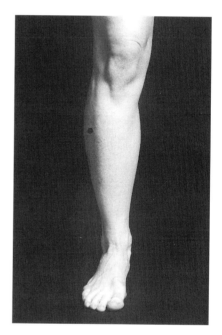

Innervation

Innervation is via the deep peroneal nerve, common peroneal nerve, peroneal division of the sciatic nerve, sacral plexus, and roots L_5, S_1.

Origin

The extensor digitorum longus originates from the lateral condyle of the tibia, the proximal three-fourths of the medial surface of the fibula, and the interosseous membrane.

Insertion

Insertion is into the dorsal digital expansion, which also receives contributions from the extensor digitorum brevis, lumbricals, and interosseous muscles. The expansion attaches to the bases of the middle phalanges with collateral slips that attach to the bases of the distal phalanges of the toes.

Activation Maneuver

Extension of the four lateral toes activates the muscles.

EMG Needle Insertion

Insert the needle 6–7 cm distal to the tibial tuberosity and 4–5 cm lateral to the shaft of the tibia. The muscle is superficial in this location, lying between the tibialis anterior and the peroneus longus (Gray's Anatomy, 1995).

Pitfalls

If the needle is inserted too laterally, it will be in the peroneus longus, which is innervated by the superficial peroneal nerve.

If the needle is inserted too anteriorly, it will be in the tibialis anterior, which is also innervated by the deep peroneal nerve.

Clinical Comments

Neurogenic changes on needle examination may be seen with lesions of the deep peroneal nerve, common peroneal nerve, peroneal division of the sciatic nerve, sacral plexus, or L_5, S_1 roots.

Extensor Hallucis Longus

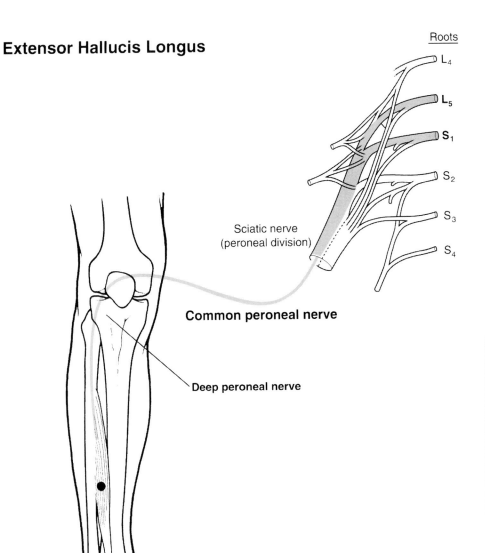

Roots

L₄

L₅

S₁

S₂

S₃

S₄

Sciatic nerve
(peroneal division)

Common peroneal nerve

Deep peroneal nerve

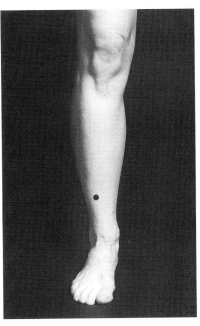

Innervation

Innveration is via the deep peroneal nerve, common peroneal nerve, peroneal division of the sciatic nerve, sacral plexus, and roots L_5, S_1.

Origin

The extensor hallucis longus originates from the midportion of the medial surface of the fibula and adjacent interosseous membrane.

Insertion

Insertion is at the base of the distal phalanx of the hallux (great toe).

Activation Maneuver

Extension of the great toe activates the muscle.

EMG Needle Insertion

Insert the needle 7–9 cm proximal to the bimalleolar line of the ankle just lateral to the shaft of the tibia.

Pitfalls

There are no pitfalls. If the needle is inserted too laterally it will be in the peroneus tertius, which is also innervated by the deep peroneal nerve; if the needle is inserted too superficial or too proximal, it may be in the tibialis anterior or extensor digitorum longus, which are also innervated by the deep peroneal nerve.

Clinical Comments

Neurogenic changes on needle examination may be seen with lesions of the deep peroneal nerve, common peroneal nerve, peroneal division of the sciatic nerve, sacral plexus, or L_5, S_1 roots.

Peroneus Tertius

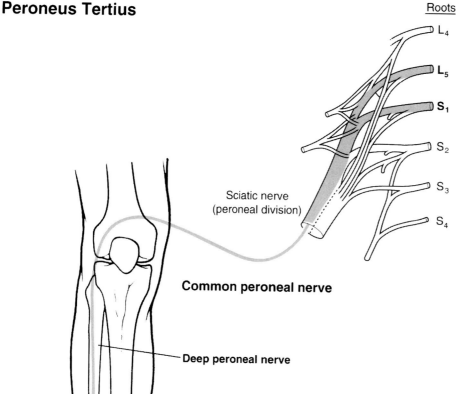

Roots

L₄

L₅

S₁

S₂

S₃

S₄

Sciatic nerve
(peroneal division)

Common peroneal nerve

Deep peroneal nerve

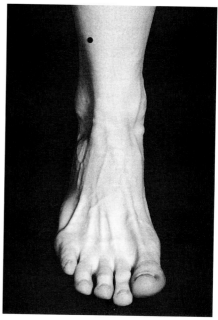

Innervation

Innervation is via the deep peroneal nerve, common peroneal nerve, peroneal division of the sciatic nerve, sacral plexus, and roots L_5, S_1.

Origin

The peroneus tertius originates from the distal fourth of the anterior surface of the fibula and the adjacent interosseous membrane.

Insertion

Insertion is at the dorsal surface of the base of the fifth metatarsal bone.

Activation Maneuver

Dorsiflexon and eversion of the foot activate the muscle.

EMG Needle Insertion

Insert the needle 6–8 cm proximal to the bimalleolar line of the ankle and 2–3 cm lateral to the shaft of the tibia.

Pitfalls

There are no pitfalls. If the needle is inserted too laterally, it will encounter the fibula; if it is inserted too anterior, it may penetrate the tendons of the tibialis anterior or extensor digitorum longus or enter the extensor hallucis longus, which is also innervated by the deep peroneal nerve.

Clinical Comments

Neurogenic changes on needle examination may be seen with lesions of the deep peroneal nerve, common peroneal nerve, peroneal division of the sciatic nerve, sacral plexus, or L_5, S_1 roots.

Extensor Digitorum Brevis

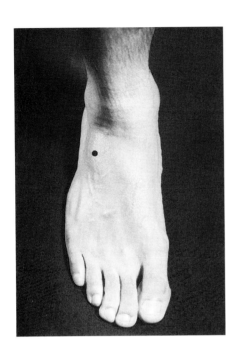

L₄
L₅
S₁
S₂
S₃
S₄

Sciatic nerve
(peroneal division)

Common peroneal nerve

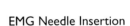

Deep peroneal nerve

Innervation

Innervation is via the deep peroneal nerve, common peroneal nerve, peroneal division of the sciatic nerve, sacral plexus, and roots L_5, S_1.

In 20%–28% of subjects, an *accessory deep peroneal nerve* also supplies this muscle (Gutmann, 1993). The accessory deep peroneal nerve is an anomalous motor branch originating from the superficial peroneal nerve. It descends on the lateral aspect of the leg, passes posterior to the lateral malleolus, and proceeds anteriorly to supply the lateral portion of the extensor digitorum brevis.

Origin

The extensor digitorum brevis originates from the anterior and superolateral surfaces of the calcaneus.

Insertion

Insertion is into the dorsal digital expansion, which also receives contributions from the extensor digitorum longus, lumbricals, and interosseous muscles. The expansion attaches to the bases of the middle phalanges with collateral slips that attach to the bases of the distal phalanges of the toes. The extensor digitorum brevis contributes four tendons; three attach to the tendons of the extensor digitorum longus for the second through fourth toes, and one inserts into the base of the proximal phalanx of the hallux; this latter slip is sometimes termed the *extensor hallucis brevis*.

Activation Maneuver

Extension of the toes activates the muscle.

EMG Needle Insertion

Insert the needle into the small mound of muscle tissue located on the proximal lateral aspect of the dorsum of the foot.

Pitfalls

The muscle may be difficult to examine in patients with peripheral neuropathies or other conditions predisposing to atrophy (e.g., compression from chronically tight shoes).

Clinical Comments

Neurogenic changes on needle examination may be seen with lesions of the deep peroneal nerve, common peroneal nerve, peroneal division of the sciatic nerve, sacral plexus, or L_5, S_1 roots.

The extensor digitorum brevis is involved early in length-dependent peripheral neuropathies.

Neurogenic changes on needle examination may reflect chronic compression of the nerve or muscle from tight shoes or high-healed shoes (Dawson et al., 1990).

This muscle is commonly used to record the compound muscle action potential during peroneal nerve conduction studies.

Peroneus Longus

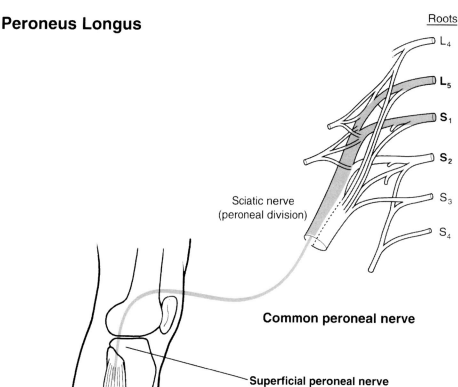

Roots

L₄

L₅

S₁

S₂

S₃

S₄

Sciatic nerve
(peroneal division)

Common peroneal nerve

Superficial peroneal nerve

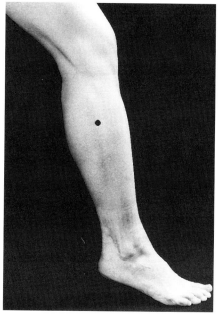

Innervation

Innervation is via the superficial peroneal nerve, common peroneal nerve, peroneal division of the sciatic nerve, sacral plexus, and roots L_5, S_1.

Origin

The peroneus longus originates from the head and proximal two-thirds of the lateral surface of the fibula.

Insertion

Insertion is at the lateral surface of the base of the first metatarsal bone and the medial cuneiform bone.

Activation Maneuver

Eversion of the foot activates the muscle. Note: This muscle can also *plantar flex* the foot because its tendon runs distally *behind* the lateral malleolus.

EMG Needle Insertion

Insert the needle 5–7 cm below the fibular head along the lateral aspect of the fibula.

Pitfalls

If the needle is inserted too posteriorly, it will be in the soleus or lateral gastrocnemius, which are supplied by the tibial nerve.

If the needle is inserted too anteriorly it, will be in the extensor digitorum longus, which is supplied by the deep peroneal nerve.

To minimize pitfalls, activation of the peroneus longus (i.e., eversion of the foot) should be performed while flexing the toes and slightly dorsiflexing the foot. This will avoid coactivation of the adjacent extensor digitorum longus and lateral gastrocnemius, respectively.

Clinical Comments

Neurogenic changes on needle examination may be seen with lesions of the superficial peroneal nerve, common peroneal nerve, peroneal division of the sciatic nerve, sacral plexus, or L_5, S_1 roots.

Peroneus Brevis

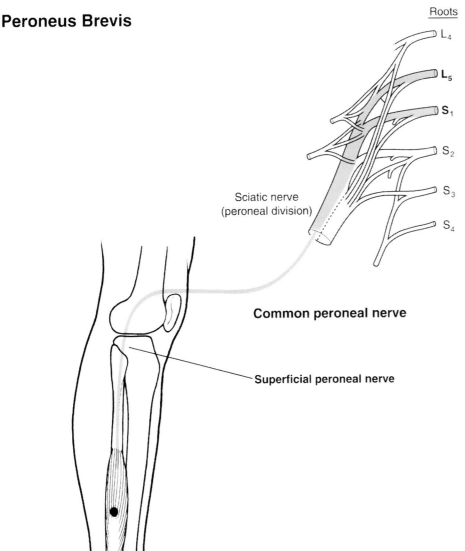

Roots

L₄

L₅

S₁

S₂

S₃

S₄

Sciatic nerve
(peroneal division)

Common peroneal nerve

Superficial peroneal nerve

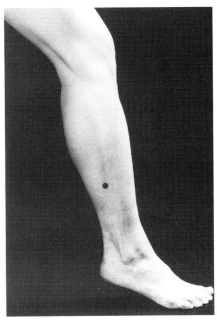

Innervation

Innervation is via the superficial peroneal nerve, common peroneal nerve, peroneal division of the sciatic nerve, sacral plexus, and roots L_5, S_1.

Origin

The peroneus brevis originates from the distal two-thirds of the lateral surface of the fibula.

Insertion

Insertion is at the lateral surface of the base of the fifth metatarsal bone.

Activation Maneuver

Eversion of the foot activates the muscle. Note: This muscle can also *plantar flex* the foot because its tendon, together with that of the peroneus longus, passes *behind* the lateral malleolus.

EMG Needle Insertion

Insert the needle 8–0 cm above the lateral malleolus just posterior to the lateral aspect of the fibula.

Pitfalls

If the needle is inserted anterior to the lateral aspect of the fibula, it will be in the peroneus tertius supplied by the deep peroneal nerve.

If the needle is inserted too deeply it will be in the flexor hallucis longus, which is supplied by the tibial nerve.

Clinical Comments

Neurogenic changes on needle examination may be seen with lesions of the superficial peroneal nerve, common peroneal nerve, peroneal division of the sciatic nerve, sacral plexus, or L_5, S_1 roots.

chapter
18

Superior Gluteal

Nerve

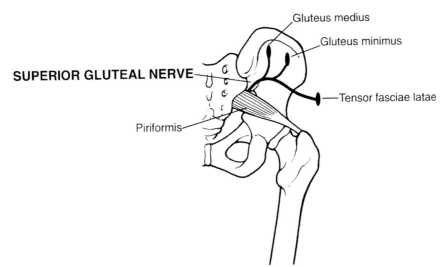

SUPERIOR GLUTEAL NERVE

Gluteus medius

Gluteus minimus

Tensor fasciae latae

Piriformis

Diagram of the superior gluteal nerve (posterior view) and its branches.

The superior gluteal nerve arises from the posterior branches of the fourth and fifth lumbar and the first sacral ventral rami. It leaves the pelvis via the greater sciatic foremen above the piriformis muscle with the superior gluteal vessels and divides into superior and inferior branches. The superior branch follows the line of origin of the gluteus minimus to supply the gluteus medius. The inferior branch crosses obliquely between the gluteus minimus and gluteus medius, distributing filaments to both of these muscles, before terminating in the tensor fasciae latae.

The gluteus medius and minimus play an essential role in maintaining the trunk upright when the opposite foot is in the swing phase of the gait cycle. In this phase, the weight of the unsupported leg tends to make the pelvis sag downward. This is counteracted by the gluteus medius and minimus of the supporting side, which exert such a powerful traction on the hip bone that the pelvis on the unsupported side is actually raised slightly (Gray's Anatomy, 1995). This supportive effect of the glutei on the contralateral pelvis depends on preserved innervation to the two muscles and on the normal relationship between the components of the hip joint. When these conditions are not fulfilled, such as in lesions of the superior gluteal nerve, congenital dislocation of the hip, or nonunion fracture of the neck of the femur, the supportive effect of the glutei is abolished and the pelvis sinks on the contralateral foot during its swing phase. This results in a characteristic lurching gait (Trendelenberg's sign). Paralysis of the gluteus medius and minimus is the most serious muscular disability affecting the hip; paralysis of other muscles acting on the hip joint produces relatively little gait dysfunction.

REFERENCES

Gray's Anatomy. 38th Edition. Churchill Livingstone, New York, 1995, pp 870–876, 1282–1288.

Gluteus Medius

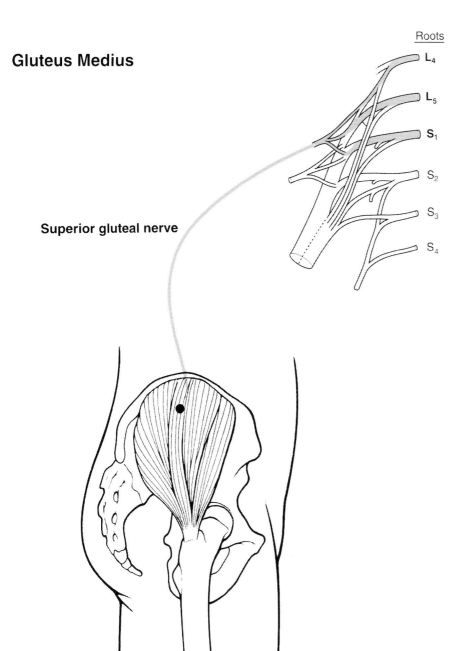

Roots

L₄
L₅
S₁
S₂
S₃
S₄

Superior gluteal nerve

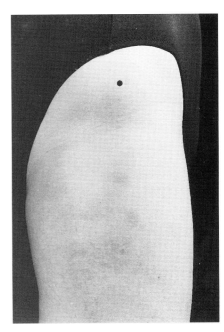

Innervation
Innervation is via the superior gluteal nerve, sacral plexus, and roots L_4, L_5, S_1.

Origin
The gluteus medius originates from the outer surface of the ilium between the iliac crest above and the anterior gluteal line below.

Insertion
Insertion is at the lateral surface of the greater trochanter of the femur.

Activation Maneuver
Abduction of the thigh activates the muscle. The anterior fibers may also contribute to medial rotation of the thigh.

EMG Needle Insertion
Insert the needle 2–3 cm distal to the midpoint of the iliac crest.

Pitfalls
If the needle is inserted too anteriorly, it may be in the tensor fasciae latae, which is also supplied by the superior gluteal nerve and L_4, L_5, and S_1 roots.

If the needle is inserted too posteriorly, it may be in the gluteus maximus, which is supplied by the inferior gluteal nerve and L_5, S_1, and S_2 roots. The posterior third of the gluteus medius is covered by the gluteus maximus.

Clinical Comments
Neurogenic changes on needle examination may be seen with lesions of the superior gluteal nerve, sacral plexus, or L_4, L_5, S_1 roots.

This is a good muscle to study for suspected L_4 or L_5 radiculopathy, because these roots primarily supply this muscle (Gray's Anatomy, 1995).

Gluteus Minimus

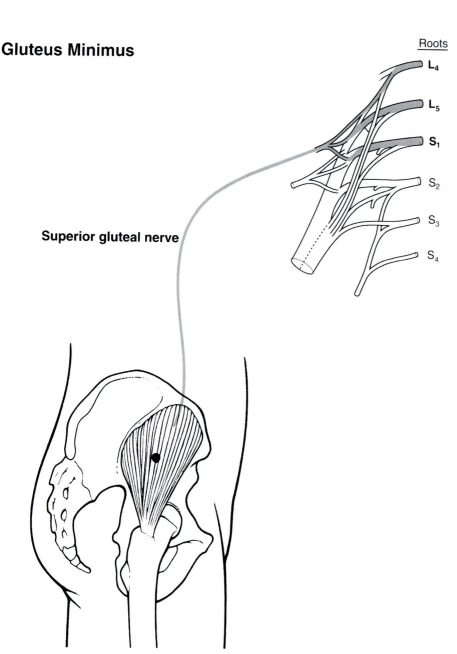

Roots

L₄

L₅

S₁

S₂

S₃

S₄

Superior gluteal nerve

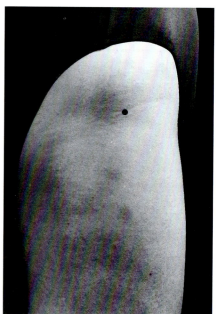

Innervation
Innervation is via the superior gluteal nerve, sacral plexus, and roots L₄, L₅, S₁.

Origin
The gluteus minimus originates from the outer surface of the ilium between the anterior and inferior gluteal lines.

Insertion
Insertion is at the anterolateral surface of the greater trochanter of the femur.

Activation Maneuver
Abduction of the thigh activates the muscle. The anterior fibers may also contribute to medial rotation of the thigh.

EMG Needle Insertion
Insert the needle midway between the iliac crest and the greater trochanter of the femur.
Insert to the bone and withdraw slightly.

Pitfalls
There are no pitfalls. If the needle is inserted too superficially, it may be in the gluteus medius, which is also supplied by the superior gluteal nerve and L₄, L₅, and S₁ roots.

Clinical Comments
Neurogenic changes on needle examination may be seen with lesions of the superior gluteal nerve, sacral plexus, or L₄, L₅, S₁ roots.
This is a good muscle to study for suspected L₄ or L₅ radiculopathy because these roots primarily supply this muscle (Gray's Anatomy, 1995).

Tensor Fasciae Latae

Superior gluteal nerve

Roots
L₄
L₅
S₁
S₂
S₃
S₄

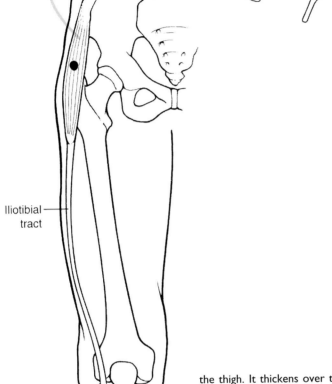

Iliotibial
tract

Innervation
Innervation is via the superior gluteal nerve, sacral plexus, and roots L_4, L_5, S_1.

Origin
The tensor fasciae latae originates from the anterior superior iliac spine and the outer lip of the iliac crest.

Insertion
Insertion is at the iliotibial tract of the fascia lata. The fascia lata is the deep fascia of the thigh. It thickens over the flattened lateral surface of the thigh to form the iliotibial tract. The upper end of this tract splits into two layers, enclosing and anchoring the tensor fasciae latae below the greater trochanter of the femur.

Activation Maneuver
Medial rotation of the thigh activates the muscle. This muscle may also contribute to abduction of the thigh and, acting through the iliotibial tract, it may also extend the knee with lateral rotation of the leg (Gray's Anatomy, 1995).

EMG Needle Insertion
Insert the needle midway between the anterior superior iliac spine and the greater trochanter of the femur.

Pitfalls
If the needle is inserted too medially, it may be in the rectus femoris or sartorius, both muscles innervated by the femoral nerve and L_2–L_4 roots.

If the needle is inserted too laterally, it may be in the gluteus medius, which is also supplied by the superior gluteal nerve and $L_{4,5}$, and S_1 roots.

Clinical Comments
Neurogenic changes on needle examination may be seen with lesions of the superior gluteal nerve, sacral plexus, or L_4, L_5, S_1 roots.

This is a good muscle to study for suspected L_4 or L_5 radiculopathy because these roots primarily supply this muscle (Gray's Anatomy, 1995).

Inferior

Gluteal Nerve

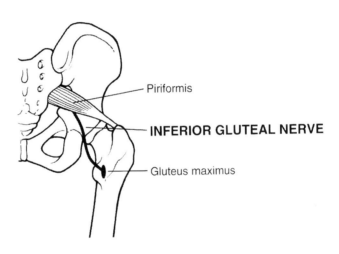

Diagram of the inferior gluteal nerve to the gluteus maximus (posterior view).

The inferior gluteal nerve arises from the posterior branches of the fifth lumbar and first and second sacral ventral rami (Gray's Anatomy, 1995). It leaves the pelvis via the greater sciatic foramen below the piriformis muscle and divides into a number of branches that enter the deep surface of the gluteus maximus. The gluteus maximus is the largest and most superficial muscle of the gluteal region. It forms the familiar prominence of the buttock.

REFERENCES

Gray's Anatomy. 38th Edition. Churchill Livingstone, New York, 1995, pp 875–876, 1282–1288.

Sunderland S: Nerves and Nerve Injuries. Williams & Wilkins, Baltimore, 1968, p 1076.

Villarejo F J, Pascual A M: Injection injury of the sciatic nerve (370 cases). Childs Nerv Syst 1993;9:229–232.

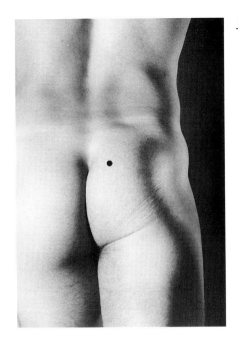

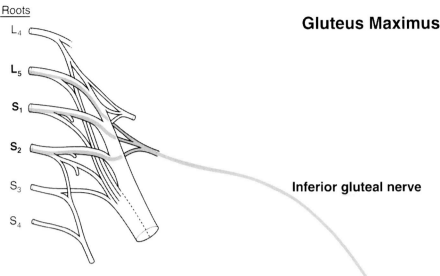

Inferior gluteal nerve

Innervation

Innervation is via the inferior gluteal nerve, sacral plexus, and roots L_5, S_1, S_2.

Origin

The gluteus maximus originates from the posterior gluteal line of the ilium and the posterior iliac crest above the line, from the aponeurosis of the erector spinae, from the lower part of the sacrum and the side of the coccyx, and from the sacrotuberous ligament and the guteal fascia that covers the gluteus medius.

Insertion

Insertion is at the iliotibial tract of the fascia lata and the gluteal tuberosity of the femur. The fascia lata is the deep fascia of the thigh. It thickens over the flattened lateral surface of the thigh to form the iliotibial tract.

Activation Maneuver

Extension of the thigh with the knee flexed activates the muscle. The patient can also be asked to contract or tighten the buttock muscles. The gluteus maximus contributes to external rotation of the thigh and, acting through the iliotibial tract, stabilizes the femur on the tibia (Gray's Anatomy, 1995).

EMG Needle Insertion

Insert the needle inside an imaginary right triangle with the hypotenuse of the tri-

Posterior superior iliac spine underlying sacral dimple

Natal cleft

angle formed by a line connecting the posterior superior iliac spine (underlying the sacral dimple) and the commencement of the natal cleft (corresponding to the third sacral spine). This will avoid the sciatic nerve, which exits the pelvis more laterally and inferiorly below the piriformis and descends between the greater trochanter and ischial tuberosity.

Pitfalls

If the needle is inserted too laterally and inferiorly, it may encounter the sciatic nerve. Sciatic neuropathy from direct needle injury or associated hematoma is a potential complication (Sunderland, 1968; Villarejo and Pascual, 1993). It is therefore prudent to avoid needle examination of that portion of gluteus maximus that overlies the sciatic nerve. (Avoid the region below the piriformis and between the greater trochanter and ischial tuberosity. Muscles in this region

Iliotibial tract

intimately associated with the sciatic nerve include the gemellus superior and inferior, obturator internus, and quadratus femoris.)

Clinical Comments

Neurogenic changes on needle examination may be seen with lesions of the inferior gluteal nerve, sacral plexus, or L_5, S_1, S_2 roots.

This is a good muscle to study for suspected L_5 or S_1 radiculopathy because these roots primarily supply this muscle (Gray's Anatomy, 1995).

chapter
20

Pudendal

Nerve

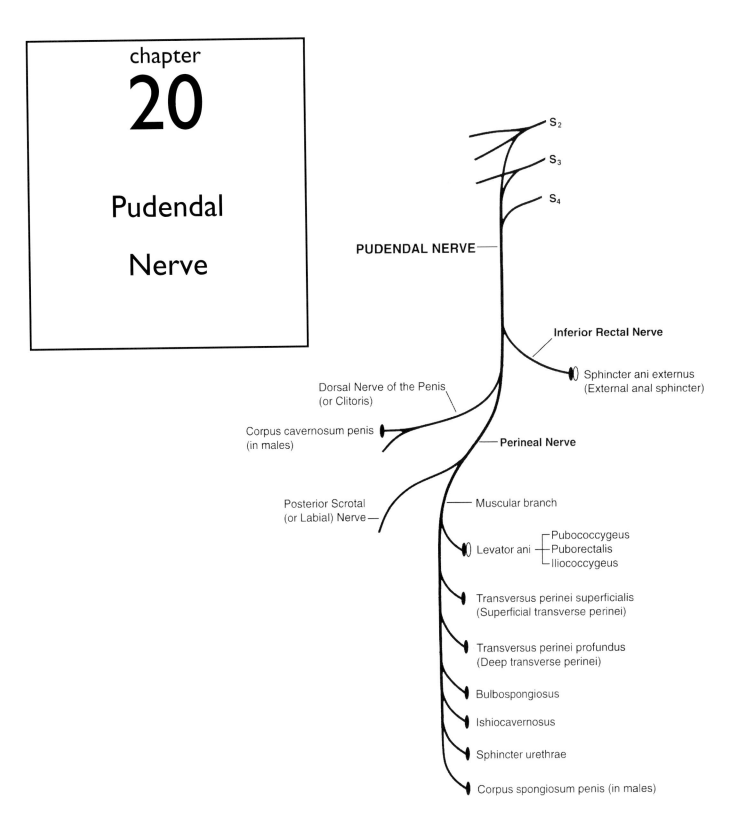

S₂
S₃
S₄

PUDENDAL NERVE

Inferior Rectal Nerve

Sphincter ani externus
(External anal sphincter)

Dorsal Nerve of the Penis
(or Clitoris)

Corpus cavernosum penis
(in males)

Perineal Nerve

Posterior Scrotal
(or Labial) Nerve

Muscular branch

Levator ani ⎡ Pubococcygeus
            ⎢ Puborectalis
            ⎣ Iliococcygeus

Transversus perinei superficialis
(Superficial transverse perinei)

Transversus perinei profundus
(Deep transverse perinei)

Bulbospongiosus

Ishiocavernosus

Sphincter urethrae

Corpus spongiosum penis (in males)

Diagram of the pudendal nerve and its branches.
NOTE: The white ovals signify that a muscle receives part of its innervation via direct branches from the sacral plexus.

The pudendal nerve is the direct continuation of the lower band of the sacral plexus and is derived from the second, third, and fourth sacral ventral rami. It leaves the pelvis via the greater sciatic foramen below the piriformis to enter the gluteal region. It then crosses the spine of the ischium and re-enters the pelvis through the lesser sciatic foramen. It accompanies the internal pudendal artery through the lesser sciatic foramen, passing into the pudendal canal (Alcock's canal) on the lateral wall of the ischiorectal fossa. In the posterior part of the canal it gives off the inferior rectal nerve. It then divides into two terminal branches, the perineal nerve and the dorsal nerve of the penis (or clitoris). In about 20% of subjects, the inferior rectal nerve arises directly from the sacral plexus (Gray's Anatomy, 1995).

The *inferior rectal nerve* pierces the medial wall of the pudendal canal, crosses the ischiorectal fossa with the inferior rectal vessels, and supplies the sphincter ani externus (external anal sphincter), the lining of the lower part of the anal canal, and the skin around the anus. The *perineal nerve*, the inferior and larger terminal branch of the pudendal nerve, runs forward with the perineal artery, dividing into posterior scrotal (or labial) nerve and muscular branches. The posterior scrotal or labial nerve connects with cutaneous branches of the inferior rectal nerve and posterior femoral cutaneous nerve to supply scrotal or labial skin. The muscular branches supply the anterior portions of the levator ani and the external anal sphincter, transversus perinei superficialis (superficial transverse perinei), transversus perinei profundus (deep transverse perinei), bulbospongiosus, ischiocavernosus, and sphincter urethrae. In males, a branch also supplies the corpus spongiosum penis. The muscles of the pelvic floor, in particular the levator ani, also receive direct innervation from branches of the second, third, and fourth sacral nerves. This is an important concept because pudendal nerve injury does not necessarily cause dysfunction in the muscles of the pelvic floor (Retzky et al., 1996). The *dorsal nerve of the penis* is the deepest division of the pudendal nerve. It supplies the corpus cavernosum penis and passes forward to provide sensation to the dorsum of the penis. In females the homologous *dorsal nerve of the clitoris* is very small.

Electrophysiologically, the muscles of the pelvic floor differ from most other skeletal muscles in that they exhibit constant EMG activity except during voiding and defecation (Retzky et al., 1996). The tonic activity in these muscles is necessary to continually support the viscera in the pelvic cavity.

Injury to the muscles or nerves of the pelvic floor often occurs during parturition. A tear involving the perineal body and perivaginal musculature may result in uterovaginal prolapse. This may often be prevented by incising the perineum (episiotomy) to provide a clean, easily reparable wound. Fecal incontinence due to anal sphincter damage or to a rectovaginal fistula may also occur following vaginal delivery or extension of a midline episiotomy (Fleshman, 1996).

PUDENDAL NERVE LESION

Etiology
Vaginal delivery (usually associated with third or fourth degree perineal tears) can cause a pudendal nerve lesion.

Pelvic tumors, including the delayed effects of pelvic radiation therapy, can be causative.

Other causes of pudendal nerve lesions are *(1)* iatrogenic (pelvic surgery),

(2) blunt pelvic trauma or penetrating injures, *(3)* compression of the perineal branches during bicycle riding, and *(4)* chronic stretch injury, usually seen with repeated and excessive straining during defecation (Dominguez and Saclarides, 1996).

General Comments

The most common cause of injury to the pudendal nerve or to its branches is parturition. Damage occurs by mechanical disruption of muscle fibers or disruption of the innervation to skeletal muscle.

Conus medullaris or cauda equina injury may damage the anterior horn cells or sacral roots, which are the source of the pudendal nerve and sacral nerves that supply muscles of the pelvic floor.

Clinical Features

Fecal incontinence can occur due to anal sphincter disruption during delivery (often associated with extension of a midline episiotomy).

Passage of flatus or stool through the vagina (rectovaginal fistula) can occur due to obstetric injury.

Numbness or loss of sensation can occur in the perineal region.

Vaginal vault prolapse may be related to partial denervation of pelvic floor muscles during delivery (Timmons and Addison, 1996).

Impotence can occur. The bulbospongiosus assists in penile erection by compressing erectile tissue of the bulb and by compressing the deep dorsal vein of the penis. The ischiocavernosus maintains penile erection by compressing the crus penis.

Urinary incontinence can occur. The sphincter urethrae surrounds not only the lower urethra but also the bladder neck. It compresses the urethra, particularly when the bladder is full, to voluntarily delay voiding.

Weakness and atrophy of the muscles of the pelvic floor occur, resulting in loss of support of the viscera in the pelvic cavity.

Electrodiagnostic Strategy

Use nerve conduction studies (pudendal nerve terminal motor latency) to evaluate a lesion of the pudendal nerve or its branches. Techniques have been developed for recording terminal motor latencies from both the inferior rectal branch and the perineal branch (Benson and Brubaker, 1996).

Pudendal somatosensory evoked potentials can evaluate pudendal sensory pathways.

Perform EMG needle examination in muscles innervated by the pudendal nerve or its branches. In pudendal nerve lesions associated with loss of motor fibers, EMG may show neurogenic changes (i.e., fibrillation potentials, polyphasic motor unit potentials, and neurogenic recruitment).

If EMG of the pelvic floor muscles is abnormal and if the etiology is not clearly obstetric, study the muscles innervated by other sacral roots to exclude cauda equina or sacral root involvement (i.e., abductor hallucis, medial gastrocnemius, and paraspinal muscles).

REFERENCES

Benson J T, Brubaker L: Electrodiagnostic assessment: A diagnostic adjunct. In Brubaker L T, Saclarides T J (eds). The Female Pelvic Floor: Disorders of Function and Support. F A Davis, Philadelphia, 1996, pp 100–108.

Dominguez J M, Saclarides T J: Preprolapse syndromes. In Brubaker L T, Saclarides T J (eds). The Female Pelvic Floor: Disorders of Function and Support. F A Davis, Philadelphia, 1996, pp 283–288.

Fleshman J W: Fecal incontinence: Etiology and evaluation. In Brubaker L T, Saclarides T J (eds). The Female Pelvic Floor: Disorders of Function and Support. F A Davis, Philadelphia, 1996, pp 208–213.

Gray's Anatomy. 38th Edition. Churchill Livingstone, New York, 1995, pp. 830–835, 1780–1782.

Retzky S S, Rogers R M Jr, Richardson A C: Anatomy of female pelvic support. In: Brubaker L T, Saclarides T J (Eds). The Female Pelvic Floor: Disorders of Function and Support. F A davis, Philadelphia, 1996, pp 3–21.

Timmons M C, Addison W A: Vaginal vault prolapse. In Brubaker L T, Saclarides T J (eds). The Female Pelvic Floor: Disorders of Function and Support. F A Davis, Philadelphia, 1996, pp 262–268.

Sphincter Ani Externus
(External Anal Sphincter)

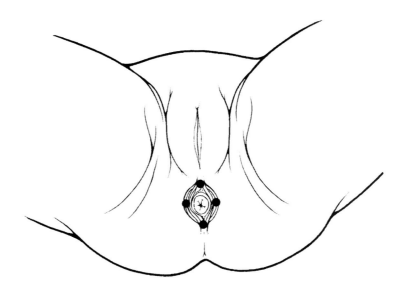

Innervation

Innervation is via the inferior rectal branch, pudendal nerve, sacral plexus, and roots S_2, S_3.

There is also, a direct branch from the sacral plexus and root S_4.

Origin

The external anal sphincter is a tube of skeletal muscle with deep, superficial, and subcutaneous layers that surround the whole anal canal.

Insertion

Fibers from deep, superficial, and subcutaneous parts attach anteriorly to the perineal body and posteriorly to the coccyx.

Some fibers blend with the puborectalis or attach to the superficial transverse perineal muscles and to the anococcygeal raphe.

Activation Maneuver

This muscle exhibits constant EMG activity that keeps the anal canal closed except during defecation. To assess spontaneous activity such as fibrillation potentials, ask the subject to bear down as if having a bowel movement. To maximally activate the muscle, ask the subject to tighten or contract the anal sphincter.

EMG Needle Insertion

Insert the needle into the external anal sphincter at the 12:00, 3:00, 6:00 and 9:00 clock positions with the patient in the lithotomy position. This evaluation should ideally be performed with the gynecological surgeon present, particularly if surgery is planned to repair mechanical disruption of the muscle fibers or disruption of the innervation to the muscle.

The presence or absence of insertional activity in different segments of the muscle (reflecting the presence or absence of viable skeletal muscle) and the inability to voluntarily contract portions of the muscle are crucial information for the surgeon.

Pitfalls

There are no pitfalls. The examiner should *not* insert his or her finger into the anus to guide the needle examination. This practice is unnecessary and poses a risk of needle injury to the examiner.

Clinical Comments

Neurogenic changes on needle examination may be seen with lesions of the inferior rectal nerve, pudendal nerve, sacral plexus, or S_2, S_3, S_4 roots.

Levator Ani

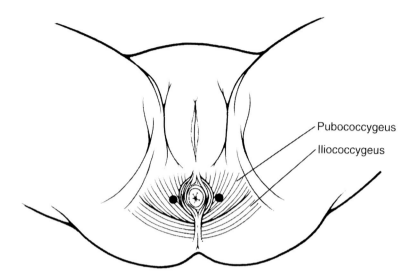

Pubococcygeus
Iliococcygeus

Innervation

Anteromedial portion: Innervation is via the perineal nerve, pudendal nerve, sacral plexus, and roots S_2, S_3, S_4.

Posterolateral portion: Innervation is via the direct branches from sacral plexus, and roots S_2, S_3, S_4.

Origin

The levator ani is a broad muscular sheet that forms the floor of the pelvic cavity. Right and left counterparts unite to support the viscera in this cavity and to surround the various structures that pass through it. The levator ani is separated into three muscular parts: pubococcygeal part (pubococcygeus), puborectal part (puborectalis), and iliococcygeal part (iliococcygeus).

The pubococcygeus arises from the back of the body of the pubis and passes back horizontally. The fibers form part of the periurethral, perivaginal, and perirectal musculature.

The puborectalis arises from the back of the body of the pubis (inseparable from the pubococcygeus at its origin) and joins its fellow muscle from the opposite side

to form a sling around the anorectal junction.

The iliococcygeus arises from the obturator fascia between the obturator canal and the ischial spine.

Insertion

Most fibers of the pubococcygeus attach to the anterior surface of the coccyx. Some fibers insert into the walls of the vagina, perineal body, and rectum.

The puborectalis joins its fellow muscle from the opposite side to form a sling around the anorectal junction.

The iliococcygeus attaches to the sides of the last two segments of the coccyx.

Activation Maneuver

Muscles exhibit constant EMG activity and contribute to bowel and bladder continence; they must relax to permit voiding and defecation (Retzky et al., 1996). To assess spontaneous activity such as fibrillation potentials, ask the subject to bear down as if having a bowel movement. To maximally activate the muscle (particularly the puborectalis), ask the subject to tighten the anal sphincter.

EMG Needle Insertion

Puborectalis: Insert the needle into the posterior half of the external anal sphincter to a depth of 2–3 cm. The puborectalis lies deep to the external anal sphincter and is separated from it by a thin layer of fat and connective tissue that results in loss of insertional activity on needle examination.

Pubococcygeus: Insert the needle 1–2 cm on either side of the external anal sphincter. The pubococcygeus is the only muscle encountered.

Iliococcygeus: This muscle is thin, aponeurotic, and not easily accessible by routine needle examination.

Pitfalls

If the needle is inserted too deeply, it may penetrate the rectum and peritoneum.

Clinical Comments

Neurogenic changes on needle examination may be seen with lesions of the perineal nerve, pudendal nerve, sacral plexus, or S_2, S_3, S_4 roots.

chapter

21

Lumbar

Plexus

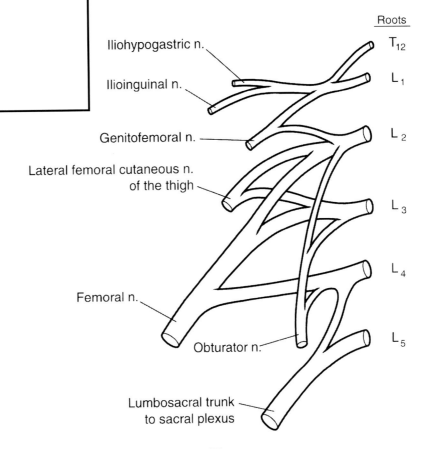

Roots

Iliohypogastric n.

Ilioinguinal n.

Genitofemoral n.

Lateral femoral cutaneous n. of the thigh

Femoral n.

Obturator n.

Lumbosacral trunk to sacral plexus

T_{12}

L_1

L_2

L_3

L_4

L_5

Diagram of the lumbar plexus (anterior view) and its branches.

The lumbar plexus is formed by the first three and most of the fourth lumbar ventral rami; the smaller branch of the fourth joins the fifth as the *lumbosacral trunk*, which joins the sacral plexus (see chapter 14). Although the fourth lumbar ventral ramus is most often divided between the two plexuses, in a *prefixed* plexus the third may be the divided ramus whereas in a *postfixed* plexus the fifth ramus contributes to both plexuses. These variations modify the lumbar and sacral plexuses (Gray's Anatomy, 1995).

The lumbar ventral rami descend laterally into the psoas major muscle to form the lumbar plexus. In its usual arrangement, the first lumbar ventral ramus, often joined by a branch from the twelfth thoracic, bifurcates into upper and lower parts. The upper part divides again into *iliohypogastric* and *ilio-inguinal* nerves; the lower unites with a branch of the second lumbar ramus to form the *genitofemoral* nerve. The remainder of the second and third and part of the fourth lumbar ventral rami joining the plexus divide into ventral (anterior) and dorsal (posterior) divisions. The anterior division of the second to fourth ventral rami form the *obturator* nerve. The posterior division of the second to fourth ventral rami form the *femoral* nerve. Posterior branches of the second and third ventral rami also form the *lateral femoral cutaneous* nerve of the thigh. Muscular branches of the lumbar plexus directly supply the quadratus lumborum, psoas minor, psoas major, and iliacus (the latter also receives innervation from the femoral nerve). The *iliohypogastric* nerve contributes innervation to the transversus abdominis and to the internal and external oblique muscles. It then supplies cutaneous sensation to the posterolateral gluteal skin and the suprapubic skin. The *ilio-inguinal* nerve also contributes innervation to the transversus abdominis and internal oblique muscles. It traverses the inguinal canal and emerges from the superficial inguinal ring to supply the proximomedial skin of the thigh and the skin covering the penile root and upper scrotm or that covering the moms pubis and the adjoining labium majus. The genital branch of the *genitofemoral* nerve supplies the cremaster muscle and provides cutaneous innervation to the scrotal skin in men or to the moms pubis and labium majus in women. The femoral branch supplies the skin over the upper part of the femoral triangle. Injury to the iliohypogastric, ilio-inguinal, and genitofemoral nerves is almost always the result of direct trauma, usually related to surgery (inguinal herniorrhaphy or retrocaecal appendix).

The *lateral femoral cutaneous* nerve of the thigh descends behind the inguinal ligament about 1 cm medial to the anterior superior iliac spine. It divides into anterior and posterior branches, the former supplying skin over the anterior and lateral thigh as far as the knee and the latter supplying skin on the lateral surface of the thigh from the greater trochanter to about midthigh. A lesion of the lateral femoral cutaneous nerve, usually due to compression behind the inguinal ligament, produces impaired sensation with pain and paraesthesias on the anterior and lateral aspects of the thigh. This condition is known clinically as *meralgia paraesthetica*.

A lesion of the lumbar plexus produces a clinical picture similar to that seen with combined femoral and obturator nerve lesions, but with additional involvement of the above-mentioned branches. It is common for femoral nerve deficit to be accompanied by obturator nerve deficit (Dawson et al., 1990) because both arise within the substance of the psoas muscle. The femoral and obturator nerves are discussed individually in the Chapters 22 and 23, respectively.

REFERENCES

Dawson D M, Hallett M, Millender L H: Entrapment Neuropathies. 2nd Edition. Little, Brown, Boston, 1990, pp 313–316.
Gray's Anatomy. 38th Edition. Churchill Livingstone, New York, 1995, pp 1277–1282.

Femoral

Nerve

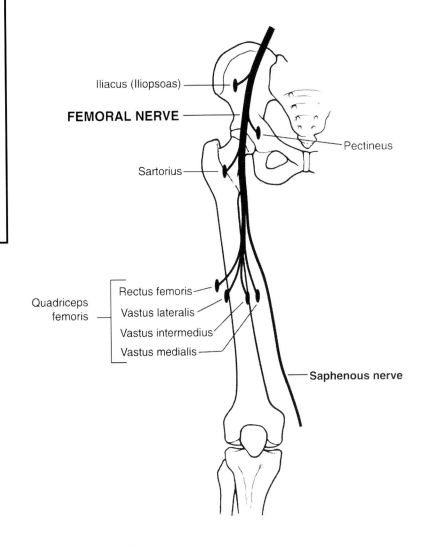

Diagram of the femoral nerve (anterior view) and the muscles that it supplies.

The femoral nerve is the largest branch of the lumbar plexus. It arises from the posterior division of the second to fourth ventral rami, within the substance of the psoas major. It emerges from the psoas at its lower outer border in a groove between this muscle and the iliacus and descends along the groove to pass beneath the inguinal ligament to enter the thigh. In the iliac fossa, it supplies small branches to the iliacus muscle (the iliacus and psoas major act together, the combination being referred to as the *iliopsoas muscle*; Gray's Anatomy, 1995). While beneath the inguinal ligament, it gives off a branch that courses medially behind the femoral sheath to supply the pectineus muscle.

Note: The short muscles around the hip joint—pectineus, obturator externus, quadratus femoris, gemellus superior, gemellus inferior, obturator internus, and piriformis—are largely innaccessible to direct observation. Because of the potential complications presented by their intimate relationship to important neurovascular structures, there is a total lack of EMG data for humans (Gray's Anatomy, 1995).

On entering the femoral triangle, the femoral nerve lies on the iliacus muscle lateral to the femoral artery. About 4 cm distal to the inguinal ligament, it divides into anterior and posterior divisions that, in turn, subdivide to give further branches. The anterior division divides almost immediately into a muscular branch to the sartorius and two cutaneous branches, the intermediate and medial cutaneous nerves of the thigh.

The *intermediate cutaneous nerve of the thigh* provides sensation to the anterior surface of the thigh as far distally as the knee. The *medial cutaneous nerve of the thigh* innervates the medial and anteromedial aspects of the thigh and continues on to innervate the medial aspect of the leg just below the knee. The posterior division immediately divides into the saphenous branch and muscular branches. The *saphenous nerve* descends to the knee where it becomes subcutaneous. It joins the saphenous vein, which it accompanies down the medial aspect of the leg. Branches of the saphenous nerve provide sensation to the skin on the medial aspect of the leg, and continue on to innervate the skin over the medial ankle and a portion of the medial foot. Muscular branches arise in spray fashion from the parent division and innervate the rectus femoris, vastus lateralis, vastus intermedius, and vastus medialis.

Anatomical features of clinical importance relate to the posterior abdominal wall, where a retroperitoneal hematoma or hemorrhage may compress the nerve (Sunderland, 1968). The appearance of signs or symptoms of a femoral nerve lesion in a patient with hemophilia or who is receiving anticoagulant therapy strongly suggests involvement of the nerve by a hematoma or hemorrhage. Compression of the nerve may also occur in this region from a benign or malignant tumor or an abscess. Beneath the inguinal ligament, the nerve may rarely be injured during inguinal or femoral hernia repair. Postsurgical femoral mononeuropathy has also been reported following positioning on the operating table in which the thigh is acutely flexed as in the lithotomy position. In these cases, nerve involvement is likely related to acute angulation across the inguinal ligament (Sunderland, 1968). In the femoral triangle, gunshot wounds and other penetrating injuries are often fatal because the femoral artery and vein are also severed. Injuries distal to the site where muscular branches arise in spray fashion result in variable involvement of the branches; some will be spared while others will be involved depending on the precise site and nature of the injury.

FEMORAL NERVE LESION

Etiology

Retroperitoneal hematomas or hemorrhages that cause a femoral nerve lesion are usually seen in patients with hemophilia or who are receiving anticoagulant therapy.

Retroperitoneal tumors (benign or malignant) and abscessess are causative.

Femoral nerve lesions can be caused iatrogenically (e.g., (herniorraphy, appendectomy, hysterectomy, femoral angiography, postanesthesia compression due to acute angulation across the inguinal ligament).

Other causes of femoral nerve lesions include (1) penetrating injuries, (2) aneurysm of the femoral artery, (3) neuralgic amyotrophy, and (4) diabetic amyotrophy (femoral nerve involvement is common).

General Comments

In diabetic amyotrophy, muscle weakness may first appear in the quadriceps muscles. Diabetic amyotrophy, however, is not simply a femoral mononeuropathy. Additional proximal muscles are involved, including gluteal, hamstring, adductor, and iliopsoas muscles (Chokroverty and Sander, 1996).

Clinical Features

The quadriceps muscles atrophy.

Paresis or paralysis of the quadriceps muscles produces weakness or an inability to extend the leg.

Paresis or paralysis of the iliopsoas, rectus femoris, and sartorius produces weakness during thigh flexion. If the iliopsoas is spared, as in a more distal lesion, loss of rectus femoris and sartorius is without noticeable effect (Sunderland, 1968).

Numbness or a loss of sensation can occur in the anterior and medial aspects of the thigh and in the medial aspect of the leg.

There is loss of the patellar tendon reflex.

Electrodiagnostic Strategy

Use nerve conduction studies (saphenous sensory response and femoral motor response) to help determine a lesion of the femoral nerve or its branches.

Perform EMG needle examination in thigh muscles innervated by the femoral nerve or its branches. In lesions associated with loss of motor fibers, EMG may show neurogenic changes (i.e., fibrillation potentials, polyphasic motor unit potentials, and neurogenic recruitment).

If EMG of the quadriceps muscles is abnormal, study other proximal muscles (gluteal, hamstring, and adductors) and paraspinal muscles to exclude plexus or root involvement.

REFERENCES

Chokroverty S, Sander H W: AAEM case report #13: Diabetic amyotrophy. Muscle Nerve 1996;19:939–945.

Dawson D M, Hallett M, Millender L H: Entrapment Neuropathies. 2nd Edition. Little, Brown, Boston, 1990, pp 313–316.

Gray's Anatomy. 38th Edition. Churchill Livingstone, New York, 1995, pp 868–875, 1277–1282.

Sunderland S: Nerves and Nerve Injuries. Williams & Wilkins, Baltimore, 1968, pp 1105–1113.

Iliacus (Iliopsoas)

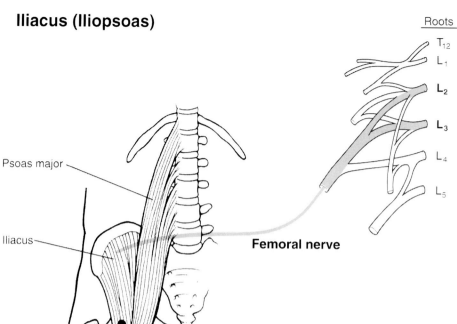

Psoas major

Iliacus

Roots

T₁₂
L₁
L₂
L₃
L₄
L₅

Femoral nerve

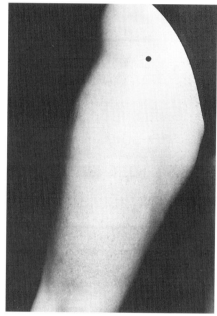

Innervation

Innervation is via the femoral nerve, posterior division of the lumbar plexus, and roots L_2, L_3. Note: Iliacus and psoas major act together, the combination being referred to as *iliopsoas*. However, direct branches from ventral rami of the lumbar spinal nerves L_1, L_2 and L_3 supply the psoas major.

Origin

The iliacus originates at the superior two-thirds of the iliac fossa, inner lip of the iliac crest, and upper surface of the lateral sacrum.

The psoas major originates at the Transverse processes and bodies of all lumbar vertebrae and the body of the twelfth thoracic vertebra.

Insertion

The iliacus and psoas major insert together into the lesser trochanter of the femur (iliacus fibers are lateral; psoas fibers are medial).

Activation Maneuver

Flexion of the thigh upon the pelvis activates the muscle.

EMG Needle Insertion

Insert the needle 3–4 cm lateral to the femoral artery pulse just below the inguinal ligament.

Pitfalls

If the needle is inserted too medially, it may penetrate the femoral nerve or artery.

Clinical Comments

Neurogenic changes on needle examination may be seen with lesions of the femoral nerve within the abdomen (retroperitoneal hematoma or mass lesion), posterior division of lumbar plexus, or L_2, L_3 roots.

Pectineus

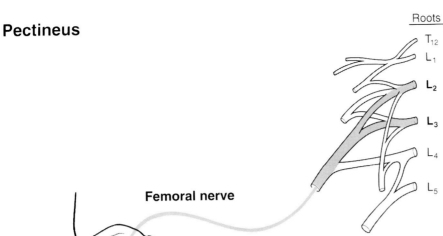

Roots
T₁₂
L₁
L₂
L₃
L₄
L₅

Femoral nerve

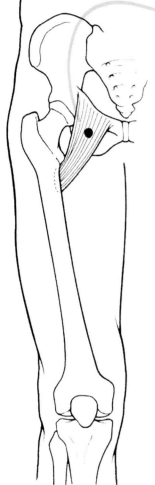

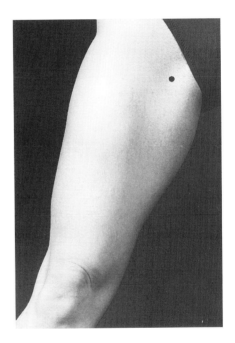

Innervation

Innervation is via the femoral nerve, posterior division of the lumbar plexus, and roots L_2, L_3. This muscle may also receive a branch from the obturator nerve (Gray's Anatomy, 1995).

Origin

The pectineus originates from the pecten pubis (superior ramus of the pubis).

Insertion

Insertion is along a line from the lesser trochanter to the linea aspera of the femur.

Activation Maneuver

Adduction and flexion of the thigh activate the muscle.

EMG Needle Insertion

Insert the needle 2–3 cm medial to the femoral artery pulse just below the inguinal ligament.

Pitfalls

If the needle is inserted too laterally, it may penetrate the femoral vein or artery; this muscle is often avoided in the EMG assessment due to its relationship with the neurovascular bundle, which traverses the lateral aspect of the muscle (Gray's Anatomy, 1995).

If the needle is inserted too medially, it may be in the adductor longus, which is supplied by the obturator nerve.

Clinical Comments

Neurogenic changes on needle examination may be seen with lesions of the femoral nerve within the abdomen (retroperitoneal hematoma or mass lesion), posterior division of the lumbar plexus, or L_2, L_3 roots.

Sartorius

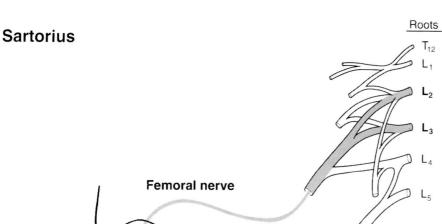

Roots

T₁₂
L₁
L₂
L₃
L₄
L₅

Femoral nerve

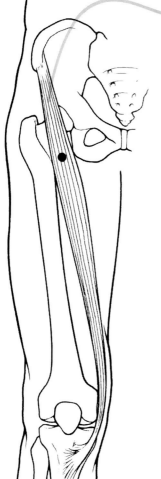

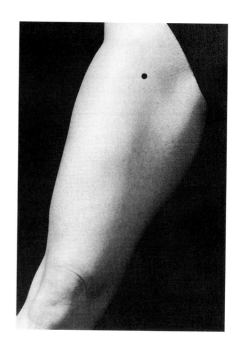

Innervation
Innervation is via the femoral nerve, posterior division of the lumbar plexus, and roots L_2, L_3.

Origin
The sartorius originates at the anterior superior iliac spine.

Insertion
Insertion is at the proximal medial surface of the tibia.

Activation Maneuver
Flexion of the thigh and flexion of the knee activate the muscle. (The sartorius is a narrow strap muscle that crosses the hip and knee joints; it is the longest muscle of the body.)

EMG Needle Insertion
Insert the needle 6–7 cm distal to the anterior superior iliac spine along a line to the medial epicondyle of the tibia.

Pitfalls
If the needle is inserted too laterally, it may be in the tensor fasciae latae, which is innervated by the superior gluteal nerve.

If the needle is inserted too medially or deeply, it may be in the iliopsoas or rectus femoris, respectively, which are also supplied by the femoral nerve.

Clinical Comments
Neurogenic changes on needle examination may be seen with lesions of the femoral nerve, posterior division of the lumbar plexus, or L_2, L_3 roots.

Rectus Femoris

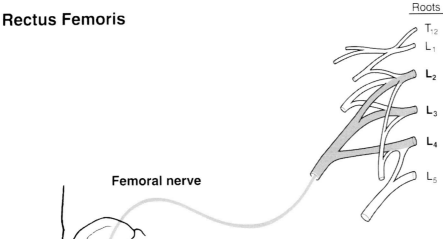

Roots

T₁₂
L₁
L₂
L₃
L₄
L₅

Femoral nerve

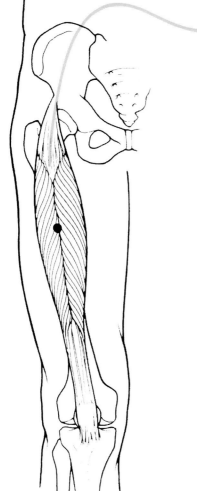

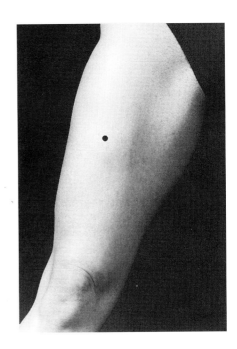

Activation Maneuver

Flexion of the thigh and extension of the knee activate the muscle. (The rectus femoris crosses the hip and knee joints.)

EMG Needle Insertion

Insert the needle into the anterior thigh midway between the anterior superior iliac spine and the patella.

Pitfalls

There are no pitfalls. If the needle is improperly inserted, it will still be in muscles supplied by the femoral nerve.

Clinical Comments

Neurogenic changes on needle examination may be seen with lesions of the femoral nerve, posterior division of the lumbar plexus, or L₂, L₃, L₄ roots.

Innervation

Innervation is via the femoral nerve, posterior division of the lumbar plexus, and roots L₂, L₃, L₄.

Origin

The rectus femoris originates at the anterior inferior iliac spine and a groove above the acetabulum of the ilium. This is the only quadriceps muscle that arises from the ilium; the other three arise from the shaft of the femur. The muscle travels straight down the middle of the thigh, hence its name *rectus femoris*.

Insertion

Insertion is at the base of the patella via the quadriceps tendon. Note: The tendons of the four quadriceps unite to form a single strong tendon attached to the base of the patella. The patella is in fact a sesamoid bone in the quadriceps tendon, and the ligamentum patellae, which extends to insert on the tubercle of the tibia, is the continuation of the tendon.

Vastus Lateralis

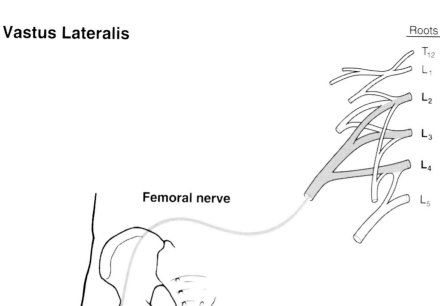

Roots

T₁₂
L₁
L₂
L₃
L₄
L₅

Femoral nerve

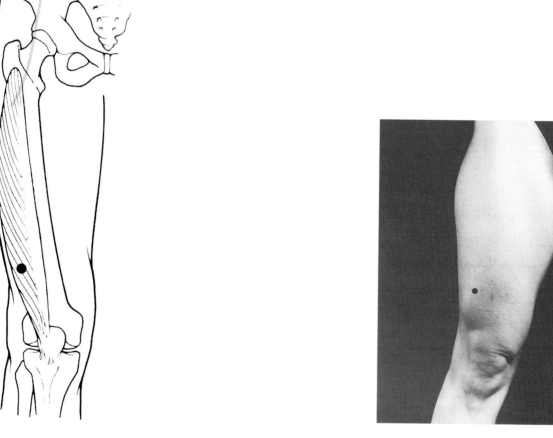

Innervation
Innervation is via the femoral nerve, posterior division of the lumbar plexus, and roots L_2, L_3, L_4.

Origin
The vastus lateralis originates from the intertrochanteric line, inferior border of the greater trochanter, gluteal tuberosity, and linea aspera of the femur.

Insertion
Insertion is at the tubercle of the tibia via the quadriceps tendon.

Activation Maneuver
Extension of the knee activates the muscle. (Instruct the supine patient to press the knee down into the bed while lifting the heel of the foot off the bed.)

EMG Needle Insertion
Insert the needle into the anterolateral thigh 8–10 cm above the patella.

Pitfalls
If the needle is inserted too posteriorly, it may be in the biceps femoris short head, which is supplied by the peroneal division of the sciatic nerve.

Clinical Comments
Neurogenic changes on needle examination may be seen with lesions of the femoral nerve, posterior division of the lumbar plexus, or L_2, L_3, L_4 roots.

Vastus Intermedius

Roots

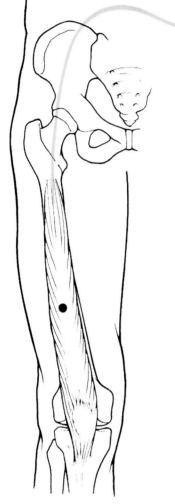

Femoral nerve

T₁₂
L₁
L₂
L₃
L₄
L₅

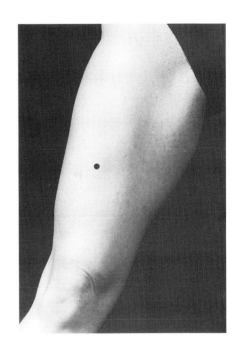

Innervation

Innervation is via the femoral nerve, posterior division of the lumbar plexus, and roots L₂, L₃, L₄.

Origin

The vastus intermedius originates at the anterior and lateral surfaces of the upper two-thirds of the femoral shaft.

Insertion

Insertion is at the tubercle of the tibia via the quadriceps tendon.

Activation Maneuver

Extension of the knee activates the muscle. (Instruct the supine patient to press the knee down into the bed while lifting the heel of the foot off the bed.)

EMG Needle Insertion

Insert the needle into the anterior thigh midway between the anterior superior iliac spine and the patella. This muscle lies deep to the rectus femoris.

Pitfalls

There are no pitfalls. If the needle is improperly inserted, it will still be in muscles supplied by the femoral nerve.

Clinical Comments

Neurogenic changes on needle examination may be seen with lesions of the femoral nerve, posterior division of the lumbar plexus, or L₂, L₃, L₄ roots.

Vastus Medialis

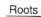

Roots

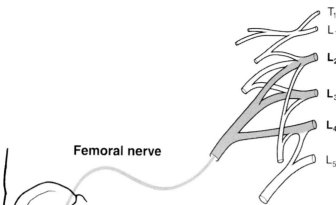

T₁₂
L₁
L₂
L₃
L₄
L₅

Femoral nerve

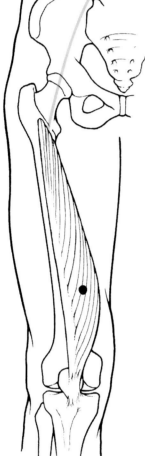

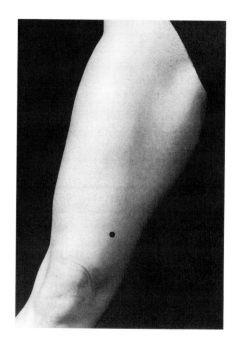

Innervation
Innervation is via the femoral nerve, posterior division of the lumbar plexus, and roots L_2, L_3, L_4.

Origin
The vastus medialis originates from the intertrochanteric line, spiral line, linea aspera, medial supracondylar line of the femur, and the tendons of the adductor longus and magnus.

Insertion
Insertion is at the tubercle of the tibia via the quadriceps tendon.

Activation Maneuver
Extension of the knee activates the muscle. (Instruct the supine patient to press the knee down into the bed while lifting the heel of the foot off the bed.)

EMG Needle Insertion
Insert the needle into the anteromedial thigh 5–7 cm above the patella.

Pitfalls
If the needle is inserted too superiorly and medially, it may be in the adductor magnus, which is supplied by the obturator and sciatic nerves.

Clinical Comments
Neurogenic changes on needle examination may be seen with lesions of the femoral nerve, posterior division of the lumbar plexus, or L_2, L_3, L_4 roots.

Obturator

Nerve

OBTURATOR NERVE

Obturator externus

Adductor brevis

Adductor longus

Gracilis

Adductor magnus

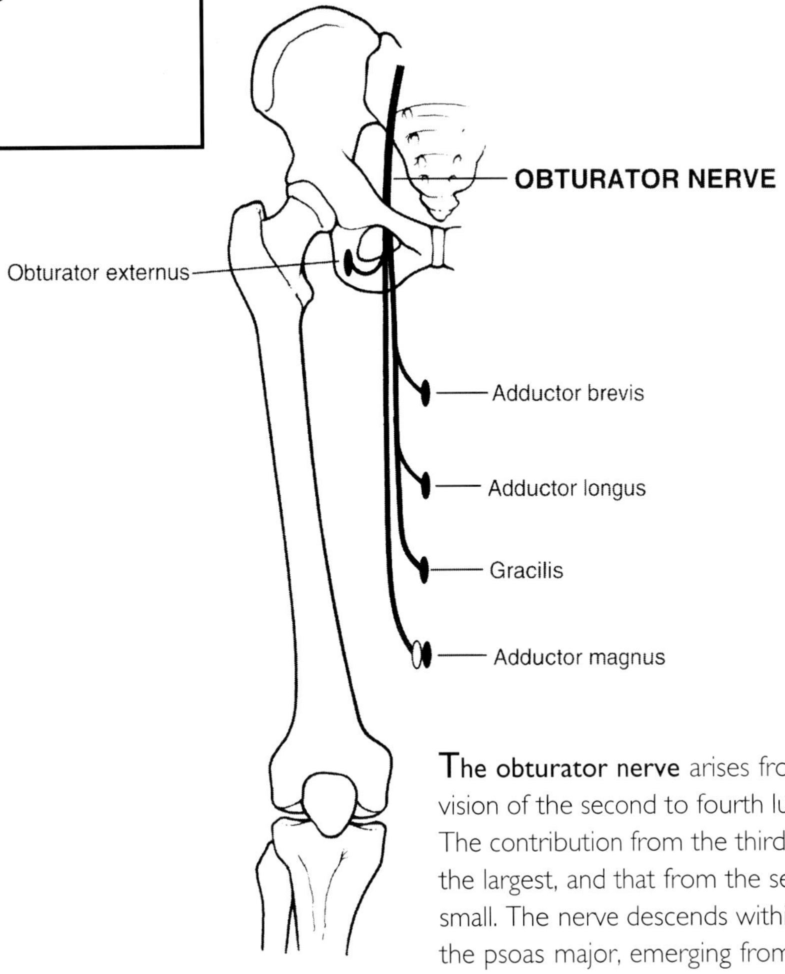

Diagram of the obturator nerve and the muscles that it supplies. NOTE: the white oval signifies that a muscle receives a part of its innervation from another peripheral nerve.

The obturator nerve arises from the anterior division of the second to fourth lumbar ventral rami. The contribution from the third or fourth ramus is the largest, and that from the second is often very small. The nerve descends within the substance of the psoas major, emerging from its medial border at the pelvic brim. It descends further along the ala of the sacrum to reach the lateral pelvic wall on the obturator internus muscle. It then sweeps forward within the pelvis to reach and pass through the obturator foramen to enter the thigh. Near the foramen it divides into anterior and posterior branches. The *anterior branch* supplies the adductor longus, adductor brevis, gracilis, and often the pectineus (Gray's Anatomy, 1995). At the lower border of the adductor longus, it communicates with the medial cutaneous and saphenous branches of the femoral nerve to supply the skin on the medial aspect of the thigh. The *posterior branch* supplies the obturator externus and adductor magnus muscles. It usually sends an articular branch to the knee joint.

A small *accessory obturator nerve* may occasionally be present, arising from the anterior division of the third and fourth lumbar ventral rami to supply the pectineus and rarely the adductor longus muscles. Note the short muscles around the hip joint—obturator externus, pectineus, quadratus femoris, gemellus superior, gemellus inferior, obturator internus, and piriformis—are largely inaccessible to direct observation. Because of the potential complications presented by their intimate relationship to important neurovascular structures, there is a total lack of EMG data from humans (Gray's Anatomy, 1995).

Anatomical features of clinical importance relate to the posterior abdominal wall, where the obturator nerve may be involved together with the femoral nerve in retroperitoneal lesions. In the pelvis, compression of the nerve may occur against the lateral pelvic wall. Here the nerve may be in direct contact with the bone or separated from it by only a thin layer of muscle (Sunderland, 1968). It may be compressed by the fetal head during a difficult delivery or by a benign or malignant pelvic tumor or abscess. On the left side it may be involved by carcinoma of the sigmoid colon and on the right by an inflamed appendix. At the obturator foramen it is intimately related to the superior ramus of the pubis, and fractures of the bone may damage the nerve. Postsurgical obturator neuropathy has also been reported following positioning on the operating table in which the thigh is acutely flexed as in the lithotomy position. In these cases, nerve involvement is likely related to acute angulation where the nerve leaves the bony obturator foramen (Sunderland, 1968). Neurectomy has been performed to relieve adductor spasms in disorders associated with upper motor neuron dysfunction.

OBTURATOR NERVE LESION

Etiology

Retroperitoneal lesions can cause an obturator nerve lesion. The obturator nerve may be involved together with the femoral nerve by hematoma, hemorrhage, tumor or abscess.

There are latrogenic causes, including neurectomy, repair of an obturator hernia, and postanesthesia compression due to acute angulation when the thigh is hyperflexed as in the lithotomy position.

Other causes include *(1)* compression of the nerve against the lateral pelvic wall by the fetal head or pelvic masses, *(2)* pelvic fractures, *(3)* penetrating injuries, and *(4)*, neuralgic amyotrophy.

General Comments

It is common for an obturator nerve deficit to be accompanied by a femoral nerve deficit (Dawson et al., 1990). Lesions of the upper portion of the lumbar plexus usually affect both the obturator and femoral nerves because both arise from within the psoas muscle.

Most lesions that involve the obturator nerve are traumatic in origin.

In diabetic amyotrophy, proximal muscles are involved, including those innervated by the obturator nerve (Chokroverty and Sander, 1996).

Clinical Features

Paresis or paralysis of adductor muscles produces weakness or inability to adduct the thigh and leg.

Numbness, loss of sensation, or altered sensation in the medial aspect of the thigh can occur.

Loss or asymmetry of the adductor tendon reflex may be observed.

Electrodiagnostic Strategy

Perform EMG needle examination in thigh muscles innervated by the obturator nerve or its branches. In lesions associated with loss of motor fibers, EMG may show neurogenic changes (i.e., fibrillation potentials, polyphasic motor unit potentials, and neurogenic recruitment).

Perform EMG of quadriceps muscles, other proximal muscles (gluteal, hamstring), and paraspinal muscles to exclude plexus or root involvement.

REFERENCES

Chokroverty S, Sander H W: AAEM case report #13: Diabetic amyotrophy. Muscle Nerve 1996;19:939–945.

Dawson D M, Hallett M, Millender L H: Entrapment Neuropathies. 2nd Edition. Little, Brown, Boston, 1990, pp 313–316.

Gray's Anatomy: 38th Edition. Churchill Livingstone, New York, 1995, pp 868–875, 1277–1282.

Sunderland S: Nerves and Nerve Injuries. Williams & Wilkins, Baltimore, 1968, pp 1096–1104.

Adductor Longus

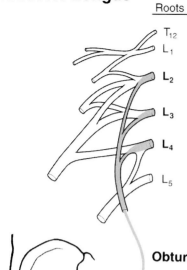

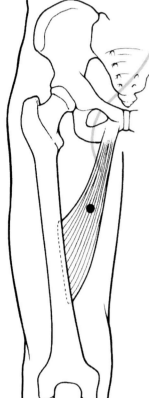

Roots

T₁₂
L₁
L₂
L₃
L₄
L₅

Obturator nerve

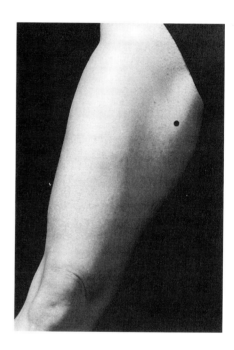

Innervation
Innervation is via the obturator nerve, anterior division of the lumbar plexus, and roots L₂, L₃, L₄.

Origin
The adductor longus originates at the front of the pubis, in the angle between the crest and the symphysis.

Insertion
Insertion is at the linea aspera in the middle third of the femur, between the vastus medialis and the other two adductors (magnus and brevis).

Activation Maneuver
Adduction of the thigh activates the muscle.

EMG Needle Insertion
Insert the needle into the medial thigh 6–8 cm distal to the origin of the tendon near the pubic tubercle. The tendon can be easily palpated.

Pitfalls
If the needle is inserted too medially and anteriorly, it may be in the sartorius, which is supplied by the femoral nerve.

If the needle is inserted too laterally, it may be in pectineus, which is supplied by the femoral nerve (the pectineus may also receive a branch from obturator nerve).

If the needle is inserted too medially or posteriorly, it may be in the gracilis or the other two adductors, which are also supplied by the obturator nerve (the adductor magnus also receives a branch from the sciatic nerve).

Clinical Comments
Neurogenic changes on needle examination may be seen with lesions of the obturator nerve, anterior division of the lumbar plexus, or L₂, L₃, L₄ roots.

Adductor Brevis

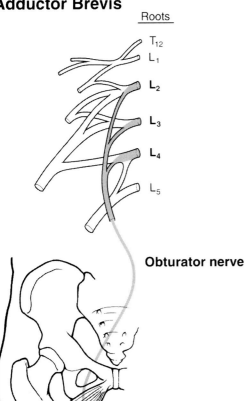

Roots

T$_{12}$
L$_1$
L$_2$
L$_3$
L$_4$
L$_5$

Obturator nerve

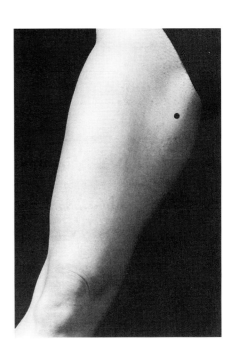

Innervation
Innervation is via the obturator nerve, anterior division of the lumbar plexus, and roots L$_2$, L$_3$, L$_4$.

Origin
The adductor brevis originates at the inferior ramus of the pubis.

Insertion
Insertion is into the femur, along a line from the lesser trochanter to the linea aspera.

Activation Maneuver
Adduction of the thigh activates the muscle.

EMG Needle Insertion
Insert the needle into the medial thigh 5–7 cm distal to the origin of the tendon of adductor longus, to a depth of about 4 cm. The adductor brevis lies deep to the pectineus and adductor longus.

Pitfalls
If the needle is inserted too superficially, it may be in the pectineus or adductor longus, which are supplied by the femoral and obturator nerves, respectively. The pectineus may also receive a branch from the obturator nerve.

If the needle is inserted too medially, it may be in the gracilis, which is also supplied by the obturator nerve.

Clinical Comments
Neurogenic changes on needle examination may be seen with lesions of the obturator nerve, anterior division of the lumbar plexus, or L$_2$, L$_3$, L$_4$ roots.

Adductor Magnus

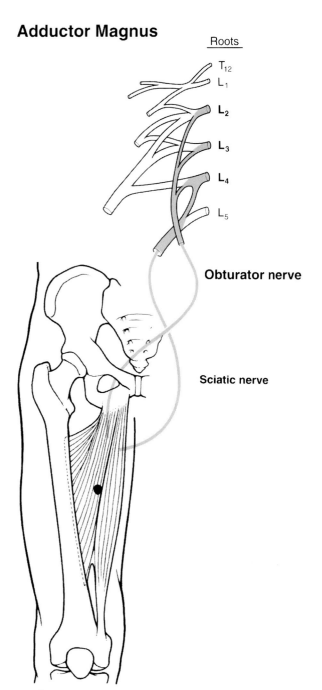

Roots

T₁₂
L₁
L₂
L₃
L₄
L₅

Obturator nerve

Sciatic nerve

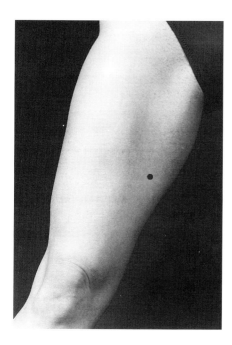

Innervation

Innervation is via the obturator nerve, anterior division of the lumbar plexus, and roots L₂, L₃, L₄.

Innervation is also via the sciatic nerve (tibial division), anterior division of the sacral plexus, and root L₄.

Origin

The adductor magnus originates from a small part of the inferior ramus of the pubis, the conjoined ischial ramus, and inferolateral aspect of the ischial tuberosity.

Insertion

Insertion is into the gluteal tuberosity, linea aspera, medial supracondylar line, and adductor tubercle on the medial condyle of the femur. The sciatic nerve supplies the ischiocondylar fibers; the obturator nerve supplies the remaining fibers.

Activation Maneuver

Adduction of the thigh activates the muscle.

EMG Needle Insertion

Insert the needle into the medial thigh midway between the pubic tubercle and medial condyle of the femur.

Pitfalls

If the needle is inserted too laterally and anteriorly, it may be in the sartorius, which is supplied by the femoral nerve.

If the needle is inserted too posteriorly, it may be in the semitendinosus or semimembranosus, which are supplied by the sciatic nerve.

Clinical Comments

Neurogenic changes on needle examination may be seen with lesions of the obturator nerve, anterior division of the lumbar plexus, or L₂, L₃, L₄ roots.

Neurogenic changes in ischiocondylar fibers may be seen with lesions of the sciatic nerve (tibial division), anterior division of the sacral plexus, or L₄ root. Morphologically, the ischiocondylar portion of the muscle may be considered to be a hamstring muscle, which explains its innervation from the sciatic nerve.

Gracilis

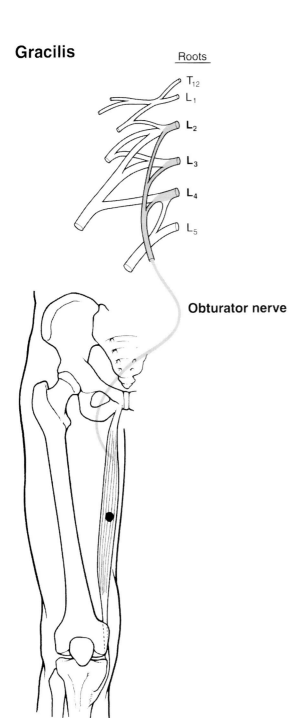

Roots

T₁₂
L₁
L₂
L₃
L₄
L₅

Obturator nerve

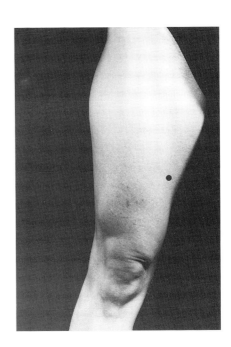

Innervation
Innervation is via the obturator nerve, anterior division of the lumbar plexus, and roots L_2, L_3, L_4.

Origin
The gracilis originates at the inferior ramus of the pubis and adjoining part of the ischial ramus.

Insertion
Insertion is into the medial surface of the tibia, just below the medial condyle.

Activation Maneuver
Flexion and medial rotation of the leg activate the muscle. The gracilis may also adduct the thigh (Gray's Anatomy, 1995).

EMG Needle Insertion
Insert the needle into the medial thigh midway between the pubic tubercle and medial condyle of the femur. The gracilis is the most superficial of the adductor group; it is thin and flat and may be missed by the needle.

Pitfalls
If the needle is inserted too anteriorly, it may be in the sartorius, which is supplied by the femoral nerve.

If the needle is inserted too posteriorly, it may be in the semimembranosus or semitendinosus, which are supplied by the sciatic nerve.

If the needle is inserted too deeply, it may be in the adductor magnus or the other two adductors, which are also supplied by the obturator nerve.

Clinical Comments
Neurogenic changes on needle examination may be seen with lesions of the obturator nerve, anterior division of the lumbar plexus, or L_2, L_3, L_4 roots.

chapter

24

Cranial

Muscles

Motor nuclei of cranial nerves VII (facial), V (trigeminal), and XII (hypoglossal) supply the cranial muscles that are most commonly tested in an electromyography (EMG) laboratory. In the caudal pons, the facial motor nucleus gives rise to the efferent fibers that form the facial nerve. This nerve supplies the muscles of facial expression, platysma, posterior belly of the digastric, and the stylo-hyoid (Gray's Anatomy, 1977). The intrapontine portion of the facial nerve initially projects posteriorly to loop around the sixth nerve (abducens) nucleus. The long intrapontine course makes it vulnerable to various brainstem lesions, which cause a peripheral rather than central type of facial palsy. The facial nerve emerges from the brainstem near the caudal border of the pons, at the cerebellopontine angle. At this site the nerve is prone to injury by acoustic neuromas or other cerebellopontine angle masses. After traversing the subarachnoid space, the facial nerve enters the internal auditory meatus. Here it begins the long and complex intraosseous course through the petrous portion of the temporal bone (facial canal). Within this segment lies the presumed site of the lesion in Bell's palsy. The facial nerve then exits the skull at the stylomastoid foramen and courses anteriorly to penetrate the superficial and deep lobes of the parotid gland. At this site the nerve is vulnerable to injury by parotid tumors and blunt trauma. Other etiologies of facial nerve dysfunction include meningitis, borreliosis, tuberculosis, herpes zoster, AIDS, and sarcoidosis. A lesion involving facial motor neurons or fibers of the facial nerve within the brainstem or in their peripheral course produces paralysis of facial movements. The particular deficit that results depends on the exact location of the lesion and its extent (for a review see Carpenter, 1976). In clinical practice, EMG of facial muscles is most commonly performed in patients with suspected Bell's palsy or in those with traumatic injury to the facial nerve.

The motor nucleus of the trigeminal nerve, located in the midpons of the brainstem, gives rise to the efferent fibers that innervate the muscles of mastication (masseter, temporalis, and pterygoids), mylohyoid, anterior belly of the digastric, and the tensor tympani and tensor veli palatini. The motor fibers emerge from the brainstem near the lateral border of the pons and exit the skull through the foramen ovale. Together with the corresponding sensory fibers, they form the mandibular division of the trigeminal nerve, which is distributed to the above-mentioned muscles. In practice, needle EMG of the muscles of mastication is most commonly performed in patients with suspected trigeminal nerve injury. Injury to the trigeminal nerve occurs with trauma (gun shot or stab wounds), surgery, infections (meningitis, borreliosis, tuberculosis, herpes zoster, and AIDS), sarcoidosis, acoustic neuromas, invasive tumors of the head and neck, and aneurysms. Clinical features of a trigeminal nerve lesion include numbness or loss of sensation over the face and weakness of closing of the jaw.

The hypoglossal nerve is a motor nerve that supplies the complex musculature of the tongue. The neuronal cell bodies that give rise to the nerve are found in the dorsal medulla of the brainstem in the hypoglossal neucleus. The nerve exits the cranium via the hypoglossal canal at the base of the skull. Injury to the hypoglossal nerve occurs with fractures of the base of the skull, tumors of the skull base, and aneurysms of the carotid artery. Hypoglossal nerve injury produces a lower motor neuron paralysis of the ipsilateral half of the tongue. Clinical signs include loss of movement, loss of tone, atrophy of muscle, and involuntary muscle twitches (i.e., fasciculations). Since the major muscle of the tongue, the genioglossus, controls protrusion of the tongue, a unilateral hypoglossal nerve injury will cause the protruded tongue to deviate to the side of the lesion. In practice, EMG of tongue muscles is often performed in patients with suspected motor neuron disease (amyotrophic lateral sclerosis).

REFERENCES

Gray's Anatomy. 15th English Edition. Bounty Books/Crown Publishers, New York, 1977, pp 299–327 and 720–756.

Carpenter M B: Human Neuroanatomy. 7th Edition. Williams & Wilkins Co., Baltimore, 1976, pp 346–349.

Frontalis

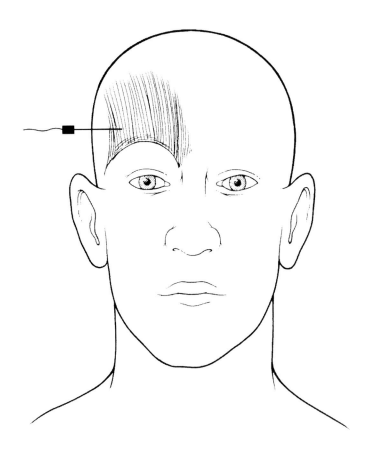

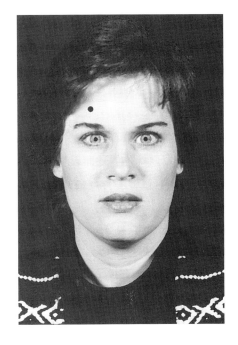

Innervation
Innervation is via cranial nerve VII (facial nerve).

Origin
The frontalis originates at the aponeurosis below the coronal suture.

Insertion
The fibers form a broad, thin, flat layer on the frontal scalp that merges with fibers from the orbicularis oculi and other facial muscles.

Activation Maneuver
Gentle raising of the eyebrows activates the muscle.

EMG Needle Insertion
Insert the needle at a 20 to 30 degree angle with the skin, 2 cm superior to the lateral half of the orbital margin.

Pitfalls
Do not insert the needle perpendicular to the skin. The muscle is very thin, and the needle must remain superficial.

Clinical Comments
Needle examination of facial muscles is usually performed in patients with suspected Bell's palsy or other injury to the facial nerve.

Neurogenic EMG changes (i.e., increased insertional activity, fibrillation potentials, excessive polyphasic motor unit potentials) occur when injury to the facial nerve or facial nucleus produces axonal loss.

Orbicularis Oculi

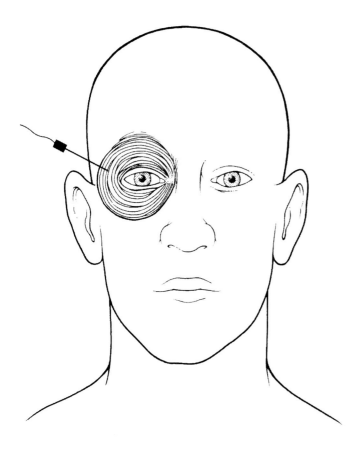

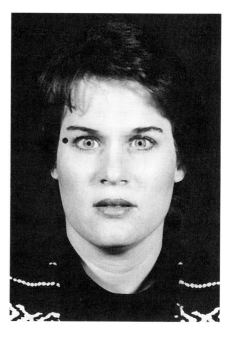

Innervation
Innervation is via cranial nerve VII (facial nerve).

Origin
The orbicularis oculi is a sphincter muscle that surrounds the orbit and eyelids (Gray's Anatomy, 1977). It arises from the frontal and maxillary bones.

Insertion
The fibers are directed outward, forming a broad, thin, flat layer that surrounds the orbit and eyelids.

Activation Maneuver
Gentle eye closure or blinking activates the muscle.

EMG Needle Insertion
Insert the needle at a 20 to 30 degree angle with the skin, lateral to the outer wall of the orbit, which is formed by the malar bone.

Pitfalls
Do not insert the needle perpendicular to the skin. The muscle is very thin, and the needle must remain superficial.

Excessive motion of the needle may result in hemorrhage ("black eye").

Clinical Comments
Needle examination of facial muscles is usually performed in patients with suspected Bell's palsy or other injury to the facial nerve.

Neurogenic EMG changes (i.e., increased insertional activity, fibrillation potentials, and excessive polyphasic motor unit potentials) occur when injury to the facial nerve or facial nucleus produces axonal loss.

Orbicularis Oris

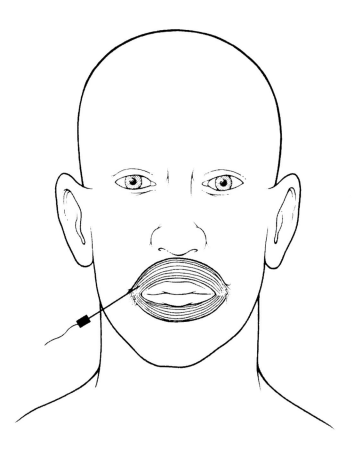

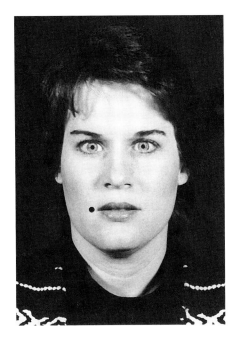

Innervation
Innervation is via cranial nerve VII (facial nerve).

Origin
The orbicularis oris consists of numerous strata of muscular fibers, having different directions, which surround the orifice of the mouth (Gray's Anatomy, 1977). These fibers are partially derived from other facial muscles that insert into the lips and partly from fibers proper to the lips themselves.

Insertion
There is no single point of insertion.

Activation maneuver
Gentle puckering of the lips activates the muscle.

EMG Needle Insertion
Insert the needle at a 20 to 30 degree angle with the skin, just lateral to the angle of the mouth.

Pitfalls
Do not insert the needle perpendicular to the skin. The muscle is thin, and the needle may penetrate the oral cavity.

Clinical Comments
Needle examination of facial muscles is usually performed in patients with suspected Bell's palsy or other injury to the facial nerve.

Neurogenic EMG changes (i.e., increased insertional activity, fibrillation potentials, and excessive polyphasic motor unit potentials) occur when injury to the facial nerve or nucleus produces axonal loss.

Masseter

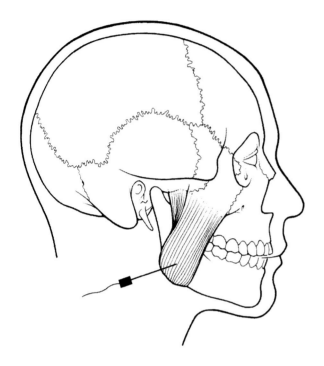

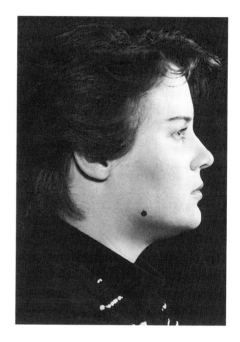

Innervation
Innervation is via the motor nucleus of cranial nerve V (trigeminal nerve).

Origin
The masseter originates from the malar process of the superior maxilla and the lower border of the zygomatic arch (Gray's Anatomy, 1977).

Insertion
Insertion is into the angle of the jaw, outer surface of the ramus, and coronoid process of the jaw.

Activation Maneuver
Jaw closure activates the muscle.

EMG Needle Insertion
Insert the needle 2–3 cm distal to the angle of the jaw and 2 cm cephalad to the lower edge of the mandible (the muscle belly is easily palpated when the patient clenches the teeth).

Pitfalls
If the needle is inserted too posteriorly, it may penetrate the parotid gland or duct that overlaps the posterior margin of the muscle.

If the needle is inserted too anteriorly, it may penetrate the buccinator muscle (supplied by the facial nerve) that lies beneath the anterior margin of the masseter muscle.

Clinical Comments
Needle examination of the masseter muscle is usually performed in patients with suspected injury to the trigeminal nerve.
Neurogenic EMG changes (increased insertional activity, fibrillation potentials, and excessive polyphasic motor unit potentials) occur when injury to the trigeminal nerve or motor nucleus produces axonal loss.

Tongue

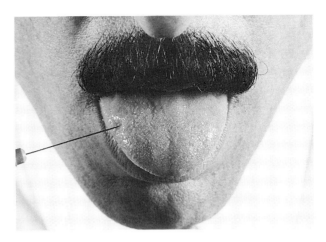

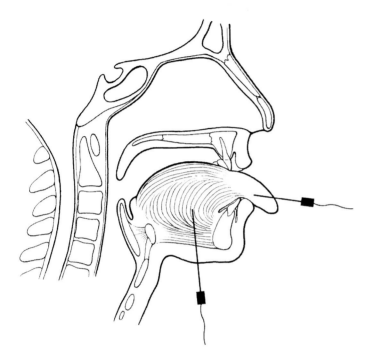

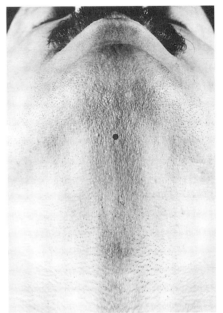

Innervation

Innervation is via cranial nerve XII (hypoglossal).

Origin

The tongue is composed of muscular fibers from multiple muscles arranged in various directions (Gray's Anatomy, 1977). This complex arrangement of the muscular fibers, and the various directions in which they run, give the tongue the ability to assume the various forms necessary for enunciating the different consonantal sounds.

The major muscle of the tongue, the *genioglossus*, arises from the superior genial tubercle on the inner side of the symphysis of the jaw.

Insertion

The genioglossus muscle spreads out in a fan-like form. The inferior fibers attach to the body of the hyoid bone, and the middle and superior fibers pass backward, upward, and then forward to enter the whole length of the undersurface of the tongue.

Activation Maneuver

Gentle protrusion of the tongue activates the muscle. Deviation away from the needle generates muscle activity.

EMG Needle Insertion

Insert the needle into the midline undersurface of the mandible 2–3 cm posterior to the tip of the chin. The needle may be angled to study the right or left genioglossus muscle.

Alternatively, the examiner can grasp the tongue with a gauze pad and insert the needle into the inferolateral portion of the tongue. To study spontaneous activity, ask the patient to gently retract the tongue so that it lies on the floor of the oral cavity.

Pitfalls

This study requires patient cooperation.

Clinical Comments

Needle examination of the tongue is often performed in patients with suspected amyotrophic lateral sclerosis.

Neurogenic changes (increased insertional activity, fibrillation potentials, and excessive polyphasic motor unit potentials) occur when injury to the hypoglossal nerve or nucleus produces axonal loss.

chapter
25

Paraspinal
Muscles

Anterior and posterior roots form the spinal nerves that exit through the intervertebral foramina. There are 31 spinal nerves on each side: 8 cervical, 12 thoracic, 5 lumbar, 5 sacral and 1 coccygeal nerve. Immediately after passing through the foramina, the spinal nerves branch into two divisions, the anterior and posterior rami.

The anterior rami form the cervical, brachial, lumbar and sacral plexuses, which in turn give rise to the peripheral nerves in the neck and upper and lower limbs. The anterior rami of the thoracic spinal nerves become the 12 pairs of intercostal nerves that supply the intercostal and abdominal muscles.

The posterior rami supply the paraspinal muscles in the cervical, thoracic and lumbosacral regions. These muscles extend the head, neck, trunk, and pelvis. Because the posterior rami branch off the spinal nerve just distal to the intervertebral foremen, needle electromyogram (EMG) abnormalities in paraspinal muscles usually imply axonal loss at the root level (i.e., radiculopathy). However, radiculopathy causes EMG abnormalities in paraspinal muscles only after structural damage or axonal loss has occurred. Hence, the

EMG may be normal when a compressing lesion irritates the root without causing axonal loss (Kimura, 1989). Moreover, the EMG in paraspinal muscles may be normal in the early stages of disease. Signs of denervation may not appear in paraspinal muscles for several days and in limb muscles for several weeks after severe root injury. Lesions limited to the plexuses or peripheral nerves do not produce EMG abnormalities in paraspinal muscles.

REFERENCES

Gray's Anatomy. 15th English Edition. Bounty Books/Crown Publishers, New York, 1977, pp 336–350.

Honet J E, Honet J C, Cascade P: Pneumothorax after electromyographic electrode insertion in the paracervical muscles: Case report and radiographic analysis. Arch Phys Med Rehabil 1986;67:601–603.

Kimura J: Electrodiagnosis in Diseases of Nerve and Muscle. 2nd Edition. F A Davis, Philadelphia, 1989, p 283.

Petrella J T, Giuliani M J, Lacomis D: Vacuolar myopathies in adults with myalgias: Value of paraspinal muscle investigation. Muscle Nerve 1997;20:1321–1323.

Cervical Paraspinal

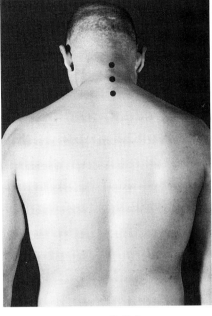

C₇ Spinous process

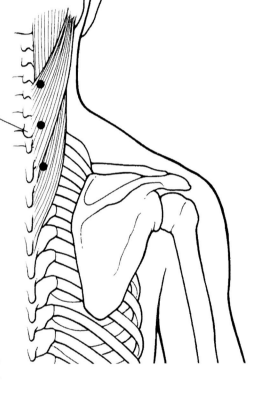

Innervation

Innervation is via the posterior primary rami of the cervical spinal nerves at the respective segmental levels.

Origin

The muscles of the paraspinal region are numerous and situated in superficial to deep layers (Gray's Anatomy, 1977). The most superficial muscles include the upper trapezius, levator scapulae, and rhomboids, with the splenius capitus and erector spinae (longissimus dorsi, transversalis colli) intermediate in depth. The deeper muscles include the multifidus, supraspinalis, interspinales, rectus capitis, and obliquus capitis, which lie deep against the vertebrae. The close proximity and overlap of the intermediate and deeper muscles makes it impossible to isolate them individually by needle examination. In general, however, the deeper muscles are shorter and receive a more discrete nerve supply from the corresponding posterior rami, whereas the more intermediate muscles are longer and receive a more overlapping nerve supply.

Insertion

It is not possible to describe all of the attachments of the muscles of the paraspinal region.

Patient Position

To achieve complete relaxation, the patient lies in the prone position with pillows underneath the chest and the forehead resting against the examining table. If full relaxation cannot be obtained, ask the patient to gently press the forehead against the table (this will cause reciprocal inhibition of the cervical paraspinal muscles).

Activation Maneuver

Ask the patient to extend the head.

EMG Needle Insertion

Identify the C₇ spinous process (the most prominent process), and count the remaining spinous processes to determine the level of the spine to be examined. Insert the needle perpendicular to the skin, or slightly upward, about 2 cm lateral to the spinous process of the desired level. The needle should encounter the lamina of the vertebra to assess the deep muscles.

Pitfalls

If the needle is too superficial, it may be in the trapezius, levator scapulae, or rhomboids.

In about 20% of thin subjects, lung tissue extends above the clavicle with a distance from skin surface to lung tissue of about 3.3 cm (Honet et al., 1986). Rarely, pneumothorax can occur following needle examination of paraspinal muscles (Honet et al., 1986). One can minimize the risk of pneumothorax by inserting the needle close to the midline, particularly when studying the lower cervical or thoracic paraspinal muscles.

The innervation to the cervical paraspinal muscles may extend one or two segments below a particular, level. This anatomical variability makes it difficult to determine the precise localization in cases of radiculopathy.

Clinical Comments

Documentation of EMG abnormalities in paraspinal muscles suggests axonal loss affecting the spinal nerve proximal to its bifurcation into the posterior and anterior rami (i.e., at the root level).

In the early stages of radiculopathy within 1–2 weeks of onset, EMG abnormalities may be limited to paraspinal muscles (Kimura, 1989); hence, EMG of paraspinal muscles is crucial in the evaluation of cervical radiculopathy.

Some systemic conditions, most notably polymyositis, may affect the paraspinal muscles preferentially and sometimes exclusively.

Thoracic Paraspinal

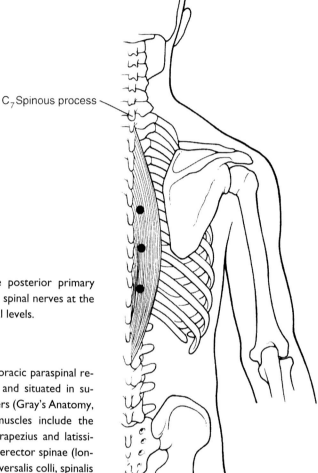

C₇ Spinous process

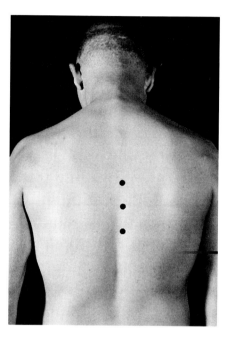

Innervation

Innervation is via the posterior primary rami of the thoracic spinal nerves at the respective segmental levels.

Origin

The muscles of the thoracic paraspinal region are numerous and situated in superficial to deep layers (Gray's Anatomy, 1977). Superficial muscles include the middle and lower trapezius and latissimus dorsi, with the erector spinae (longissimus dorsi, transversalis colli, spinalis dorsi) intermediate in depth. The deeper muscles include the multifidus, rotatores, interspinales, and semispinalis, which lie deep against the vertebrae. The close proximity and overlap of the intermediate and deeper muscles makes it impossible to isolate them individually by needle examination. In general, however, the deeper muscles are shorter and receive a more discrete nerve supply from the corresponding posterior rami, whereas the more intermediate muscles are longer and receive a more overlapping nerve supply.

Insertion

It is not possible to describe all of the attachments of the muscles of the paraspinal region.

Patient Position

The patient lies in the prone position with pillows underneath the chest and the forehead resting against the examining table. Alternatively, the patient may be flat or in the side-lying fetal position.

Activation Maneuver

Ask the patient to gently arch the back.

EMG Needle Insertion

Identify the C₇ spinous process (the most prominent process), and count down the remaining spinous processes to determine the level of the spine to be examined. Insert the needle perpendicular to the skin, about 2 cm lateral to the spinous process of the desired level. The needle should encounter the lamina of the vertebra to assess the deep muscles.

Pitfalls

If the needle is too superficial, it may be in the trapezius or latissimus dorsi.

Rarely, pneumothorax can occur following needle examination of paraspinal muscles (Honet et al., 1986). One can minimize the risk of pneumothorax by inserting the needle close to the midline.

Clinical Comments

Documentation of EMG abnormalities in thoracic paraspinal muscles suggests axonal loss affecting the spinal nerve proximal to its bifurcation into posterior and anterior rami (i.e., at the root level).

Some systemic conditions, most notably polymyositis, may affect the paraspinal muscles preferentially and sometimes exclusively (Kimura, 1989; Petrella et al., 1997).

Lumbosacral Paraspinal

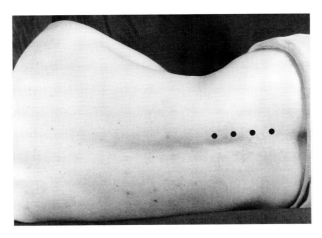

Innervation

Innervation is via the posterior primary rami of the lumbar and sacral spinal nerves at the respective levels.

Origin

The muscles of the paraspinal region are numerous and situated in superficial to deep layers (Gray's Anatomy, 1977). Superficial muscles include the latissimus dorsi, with the erector spinae (longissimus dorsi, spinalis dorsi) intermediate in depth. The deeper muscles include the multifidus and interspinales, which lie deep against the vertebrae. The close proximity and overlap of these muscles makes it impossible to isolate them individually by needle examination. In general, however, the deeper muscles are shorter and receive a more discrete nerve supply from the corresponding posterior rami, whereas the more superficial muscles are longer and receive a more overlapping nerve supply.

Insertion

It is not possible to describe all of the attachments of the muscles of the paraspinal region.

Patient Position

The patient lies in the prone position with pillows placed underneath the abdomen. Alternatively, the patient may be in the side-lying fetal position. In the latter position, the muscles on the side farthest from the table are generally relaxed.

Activation Maneuver

For the prone position, ask the patient to elevate the whole leg (perform hip extension). For the side-lying fetal position, ask the patient to perform hip extension against resistance by the examiner.

EMG Needle Insertion

Draw an imaginary line connecting the posterior superior iliac crests. This line intersects the lumbar spine at the L_3–L_4 intervertebral level. Count up or down the spinous processes to determine the paraspinal level to be examined. Insert the needle perpendicular to the skin, about 2 cm lateral to the spinous process of the desired level. The needle should encounter the lamina of the vertebra to assess the deep muscles.

Pitfalls

If the needle is too superficial, it may be in the latissimus dorsi.

To facilitate relaxation of these muscles, instruct the patient to push the small of the back against the examiner's hands.

L$_3$- L$_4$ Level

Posterior superior iliac crest

Clinical Comments

Documentation of EMG abnormalities in lumbosacral paraspinal muscles suggests axonal loss affecting the spinal nerve proximal to its bifurcation into the posterior and anterior rami (i.e., at the root level).

Some systemic conditions, most notably polymyositis, may affect the paraspinal muscles preferentially and sometimes exclusively (Kimura, 1989; Petrella et. al., 1997).

Index